T0328827

Curbside Consultation
of the Shoulder

49 Clinical Questions

CURBSIDE CONSULTATION IN ORTHOPEDICS
SERIES

SERIES EDITOR, BERNARD R. BACH, JR., MD

Curbside Consultation

of the Shoulder

49 Clinical Questions

EDITED BY

Gregory P. Nicholson, MD
Chicago, Illinois

Matthew T. Provencher, MD, LCDR, MC, USNR
San Diego, California

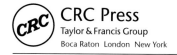

CRC Press
Taylor & Francis Group
Boca Raton London New York

CRC Press is an imprint of the
Taylor & Francis Group, an **informa** business

First published 2008 by SLACK Incorporated

Published 2024 by CRC Press
2385 NW Executive Center Drive, Suite 320, Boca Raton FL 33431

and by CRC Press
4 Park Square, Milton Park, Abingdon, Oxon, OX14 4RN

CRC Press is an imprint of Taylor & Francis Group, LLC

© 2008 Taylor & Francis Group, LLC

Library of Congress Cataloging-in-Publication Data

Curbside consultation of the shoulder : 49 clinical questions / edited by Gregory P. Nicholson, Matthew T. Provencher.
  p. ; cm. -- (Curbside consultation in orthopedics)
 Includes bibliographical references and index.
 ISBN 978-1-55642-827-2 (softcover : alk. paper)
1. Shoulder--Wounds and injuries--Miscellanea. 2. Sports injuries--Treatment--Miscellanea. I. Nicholson, Gregory P. II. Provencher, Matthew T. III. Series.
 [DNLM: 1. Shoulder--injuries. 2. Athletic Injuries--therapy. 3. Musculoskeletal Diseases--therapy. 4. Rotator Cuff--injuries. 5. Shoulder Joint--injuries. WE 810 C975 2008]
 RD557.5.C87 2008
 617.5′72044--dc22
                              2008017409

ISBN: 9781556428272 (pbk)
ISBN: 9781003523772 (ebk)

DOI: 10.1201/9781003523772

Dedication

To my wife and family for their understanding and patience; and my colleagues, mentors, and residents and fellows for their knowledge and enthusiasm, it has allowed me to be a better physician with each day.

Gregory P. Nicholson, MD

To my wife, Melissa; Connor, Brody, and my loving and supportive parents.

Matthew T. Provencher, MD, LCDR, MC, USNR

Contents

About the Editors

Gregory P. Nicholson, MD is an Associate Professor of Orthopaedic Surgery at Rush University Medical Center in Chicago, Illinois. He is an author of numerous articles, papers, and chapters on conditions and injuries on the shoulder and elbow. He is a team physician for the Chicago White Sox baseball team. He is a member of the American Shoulder and Elbow Surgeons and American Orthopaedic Society for Sports Medicine.

Matthew T. Provencher, MD, LCDR, MC, USNR was born in New Hampshire, and completed his undergraduate education at the United States Naval Academy. There, he graduated with Distinction, was inducted into Phi Kappa Phi (National Honor Society), Tau Beta Pi (National Engineering Honor Soecity), Sigma Pi Sigma (National Physics Honor Society), and was named the Secretary of the Navy Distinguished Graduate. He was also a 4-year varsity oarsman and All-American at Navy. He completed his medical education at Dartmouth Medical School where he graduated with Honors and was elected to the Alpha Omega Alpha Honor Society.

Matt completed his orthopaedic residency at the Naval Medical Center San Diego and his orthopaedic sports fellowship at Rush University under the direction of Bernard R. Bach, Jr, MD. Matt has been awarded the International Society of Arthroscopy, Knee Surgery and Orthopaedic Sports Medicine (ISAKOS) Science Award, the ISAKOS Richard Caspari Award (runner-up), the American Orthopaedic Society for Sports Medicine (AOSSM) Aircast Research Award, and was also both an AOSSM (Asia-Pacific) and an AOA John Fahey North American Traveling Fellow.

Matt is currently the Assistant Director of Shoulder, Knee and Sports Surgery at the Naval Medical Center San Diego, a full-time academic practice.

He is an active member of Arthroscopy Association of North America (AANA), AOSSM, ISAKOS, International Cartilage Repair Society (ICRS), and Society of Military Orthopaedic Surgeons (SOMOS).

Contributing Authors

Christopher S. Ahmad, MD
Columbia Orthopaedics
New York, NY

Robert A. Arciero, MD
University of Connecticut
Farmington, CT

John-Erik Bell, MD
Dartmouth-Hitchcock Medical Center
Lebanon, NH

R. Bryan Butler, MD
University of Maryland School of Medicine
Baltimore, MD

Joseph Carney, MD
Naval Medical Center San Diego
San Diego, CA

Justin W. Chandler, MD
University North Carolina Chapel Hill
Chapel Hill, NC

Joseph Y. Choi, MD, PhD
Upstate Medical University
Syracuse, NY

Alex Creighton, MD
University North Carolina, Chapel Hill
Chapel Hill, NC

Christopher Dewing, MD
Naval Medical Center San Diego
San Diego, CA

T. Bradley Edwards, MD
Fondren Orthopaedic Group, LLP
University of Texas Health Science Center
Baylor College of Medicine
Houston, TX

Michael Freehill, MD
Sports & Orthopaedic Specialists
   Minneapolis, MN;
University of Minnesota
Minneapolis, MN

Ed Glenn, MD
Tennessee Orthopaedic Alliance
Nashville, TN

R. Michael Gross, MD
Naval Medical Center San Diego
San Diego, CA

Samer S. Hasan, MD, PhD
University of Cincinnati
Cincinnati, OH

Paul Jarman, MD
The Carrell Clinic
Dallas, TX

Sumant G. "Butch" Krishnan, MD
The Carrell Clinic
Dallas, TX

Kenneth C. Lin, MD
The Carrell Clinic
Dallas, TX

G. Peter Maiers II, MD
Methodist Sports Medicine/
The Orthopaedic Specialists
Indianapolis, IN

Craig S. Mauro, MD
UPMC Center for Sports Medicine
Pittsburgh, PA

Augustus D. Mazzocca, MD
University of Connecticut
Farmington, CT

Anand Murthi, MD
University of Maryland School of Medicine
Baltimore, MD

James M. Paci, MD
Upstate Medical University
Syracuse, NY

Michael L. Pearl, MD
Kaiser Permanente
Los Angeles, CA

A. Dushi Parameswaran, MD
Rush University Medical Center
Chicago, IL

John Reineck MD
The Carrell Clinic
Dallas, TX

Clifford G. Rios, MD
University of Connecticut
Farmington, CT

Mark W. Rodosky, MD
UPMC Center for Sports Medicine
Pittsburgh, PA

Anthony A. Romeo, MD
Rush University Medical Center
Chicago, IL

K. Blair Sampson, MD
Wake Forest University School of Medicine
Winston-Salem, NC

David L. Saxton, MD
McBride Orthopedics, Inc.
Oklahoma City, OK

Matthew G. Scuderi, MD
Upstate Medical University
Syracuse, NY

Daniel J. Solomon, MD
Naval Medical Center San Diego
San Diego, CA

Rodney J. Stanley, MD
Northshore Orthopedic & Sports Medicine
   Center
Mooresville, NC

Matthew D. Williams, MD
Acadiana Orthopaedic Group
Lafayette, LA
LSU Health Science Center
New Orleans, LA

Scot A. Youngblood, MD
Medical Corps
United States Navy
Naval Hospital Pensacola
Pensacola, FL

Preface

The care and treatment of shoulder problems, conditions, and injuries is a large and diverse field of orthopaedic surgery. The knowledge base and the techniques to treat shoulder problems have rapidly expanded in the last 10 years. It can be difficult to keep abreast of the latest developments, while not losing sight of time-tested principles.

The goal of *Curbside Consultation of the Shoulder* is to provide the practicing orthopaedic surgeon, fellow, and resident concise answers to real-world clinical problems and cases that they will encounter. Authors were chosen for their experience and expertise in the subject field, as well as their practical clinical advice.

Questions were chosen throughout the scope of clinical shoulder practice. These are questions we have been asked ourselves or have asked ourselves many times in the past. There are specific clinical situations and some more general topics that impact the physician on an almost daily basis. It is hoped that this text will give the reader a guideline to help treat those patients with shoulder problems, and provide a resource to refer back to.

Gregory P. Nicholson, MD
Matthew T. Provencher, MD, LCDR, MC, USNR

SECTION I

PHYSICAL EXAMINATION QUESTIONS

QUESTION

1

WHAT ARE THE PHYSICAL EXAMINATION FINDINGS THAT LEAD YOU TO A DIAGNOSIS OF GLENOHUMERAL INTERNAL ROTATION DEFICIT IN THE THROWING ATHLETE AND WHAT NONOPERATIVE TREATMENT OPTIONS HAVE LED TO IMPROVEMENT OF THE CONDITION?

Daniel J. Solomon, MD

Glenohumeral internal rotation deficit (GIRD) is a pathologic lack of internal rotation of the throwing arm compared to the nonthrowing arm. Fortunately in the throwing athlete, the patient's nonthrowing arm usually provides a useful control to evaluate range of motion (ROM). If there is a loss of greater than 25 degrees of internal rotation of the throwing shoulder compared to the nonthrowing shoulder, the diagnosis of GIRD is made. An assumption of GIRD can also be made if the total ROM is 10% less than the nonthrowing shoulder.[1]

The diagnosis is made during physical examination of passive ROM. It is best to check internal rotation in the supine position, with the shoulder abducted. It can also be considered during an apprehension-relocation test during physical examination. Often the GIRD patient has a hyperexternal rotation when performing these maneuvers. The supine examination allows the examiner better control of scapular motion than a seated or standing evaluation. Glenohumeral motion is isolated as much as possible by pushing down gently on the anterior shoulder to eliminate as much scapular motion as possible

Figure 1-1. (A) Supine abducted shoulder position with assessment for internal rotation from a lateral view. (B) Supine abducted shoulder position for assessment of internal rotation. The examiner is stabilizing the scapula with anterior pressure.

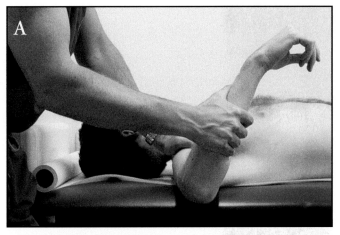

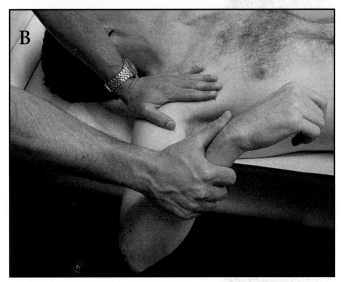

(Figure 1-1). Motion should also be evaluated with the patient seated to assess dynamic ROM. Interestingly, Myers and colleagues found that throwers with pathologic internal rotation deficits did not have increased external rotation gain compared to their asymptomatic controls; rather, both groups had similar external rotation but the symptomatic group had greater GIRD and posterior capsular tightness.[2]

Burkhart and colleagues espoused the concept that "acquired posteroinferior capsular contracture is the first and essential abnormality that initiates a pathologic cascade that climaxes in the late cocking phase of throwing."[1] They went on to elegantly describe a series of events that may subsequently occur with protracted throwing in a patient with GIRD. After the development of a tight posteroinferior capsule, when the shoulder is in a hyperexternally rotated and abducted position, the shoulder has shifted superiorly and posteriorly. This creates shear on the posterior superior labrum anterior to posterior (SLAP) region and biceps anchor. Pseudolaxity of the anterior structures develops as well. Shear and torsional stress on the rotator cuff as well as friction from the frayed labrum and internal impingement can create a partial articular sided rotator cuff tear.

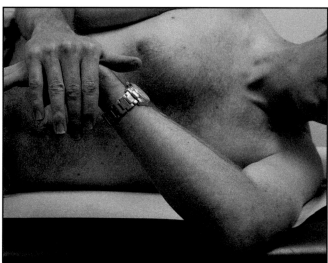

Figure 1-2. The "sleeper stretch." The patient lies on the affected side with the shoulder abducted and flexed to 90 degrees. The goal is to lie on the scapula so that it is flat on the floor or table. The patient then progressively passively internally rotates the forearm with his or her opposite hand. A modified "sleeper stretch" position can also help; the arm is in the same position of forward flexion but the patient is lying more prone using his or her body rotation to apply more adduction to the arm.

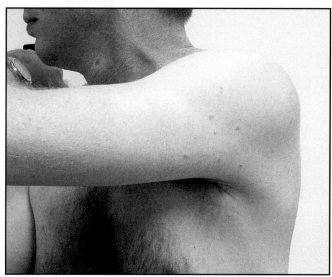

Figure 1-3. The "cross-body adduction stretch." The shoulder is held in a forward flexed position at 90 degrees and the arm is adducted across the body with the opposite hand. With a profound posterior capsular contracture, this stretch may only just move the scapula and not effectively stretch the capsule.

Furthermore, those same authors indicated excellent success with a posteroinferior capsular stretching program to reduce GIRD.[1] It is quite unusual for a younger or recreational athlete to be a nonresponder when the patient is compliant with the stretching program described (Figures 1-2 and 1-3). Wilk and colleagues described the concepts for rehabilitation of the throwing athlete and included a phased program that includes a posterior stretching program.[3] Regardless of etiology, a program to keep the posterior musculature flexible and the posterior capsule mobile has been effective in both the treatment and prevention of GIRD.[4] Additional gains can be made working with these athletes on a scapular control program that includes strengthening of the rhomboid, trapezius, and serratus anterior muscles. A rotator cuff strengthening regimen should also be initiated.

References

1. Burkhart SS, Morgan CD, Kibler WB. Current concepts: the disabled throwing shoulder: spectrum of pathology. Part 1: pathoanatomy and biomechanics. *Arthroscopy.* 2003;19:404-420.
2. Myers JB, Laudner KG, Pasquale MR, Bradley JP, Lephart SM. Glenohumeral range of motion deficits and posterior shoulder tightness in throwers with pathologic internal impingement. *Am J Sports Med.* 2006;34:385-391.
3. Wilk KE, Meister K, Andrews JR. Current concepts in the rehabilitation of the overhead throwing athlete. *Am J Sports Med.* 2002;30:136-151.
4. Lintner D, Mayol M, Uzodinma O, Jones, R, Labossiere D. Glenohumeral internal rotation deficits in professional pitchers enrolled in an internal rotation stretching program. *Am J Sports Med.* 2007;35:617-621.

WHAT PHYSICAL EXAMINATION TESTS OR FINDINGS AND RADIOGRAPHS DO YOU USE TO DIAGNOSE SUBACROMIAL IMPINGEMENT, AND WHEN DO YOU UTILIZE SUBACROMIAL INJECTIONS?

Scot A. Youngblood, MD

One of the most common shoulder diagnoses that I encounter is shoulder impingement syndrome. When I am evaluating a patient with suspected impingement syndrome, it is important to rule out other important potential concomitant shoulder pathologies. A thorough physical examination including gross inspection, range of motion (ROM), and provocative testing should be performed to exclude other causes of shoulder pain. The differential diagnosis of someone with suspected impingement includes adhesive capsulitis, calcific tendonitis, superior labral tears, biceps tendinopathy, and arthritides of the glenohumeral and acromioclavicular joints.

Subacromial impingement is often a poorly localized pain, deep-seated within the shoulder, and is exacerbated with overhead activity and shoulder exertion. I take the shoulder through gentle passive ROM testing and usually find mild loss of ROM, with the extremes of internal rotation and forward flexion being the most commonly affected. Tenderness to palpation is typically rare, but can be present at the site of supraspinatus insertion on the greater tuberosity. Provocative tests include Neer's impingement sign (pain with shoulder forward flexion and internal rotation), Neer's impingement test (pain with forward flexion relieved following a subacromial injection of anesthetic), and Hawkin's sign (pain with forced internal rotation in the 90 degree forward-flexed position). Although these tests are the most commonly used in clinical practice, my clinical practice and others have found them less than ideal. One analysis found the Neer's impingement sign and Hawkin's sign in the diagnosis of bursitis to have sensitivities of 75% and 92% and specificities of 48% and 44%, respectively.[1]

I always perform strength testing of the rotator cuff muscles in isolation to exclude complete tears. The supraspinatus is typically isolated utilizing Jobe's test (muscle testing against resistance in the 90-degree abducted, 30-degree forward-flexed, and internally rotated position). The drop sign is used to evaluate the infraspinatus (the patient holds the shoulder maximally externally rotated after the examiner releases the wrist with the elbow flexed 90 degrees and the shoulder flexed 90 degrees in the scapular plane). Finally, the subscapularis is evaluated for integrity with the lift-off test (the patient lifts the dorsum of the hand off the small of his or her back with the shoulder internally rotated) as well as the belly press test (holding hand internally rotated against the abdomen, with full resistance). If I suspect a complete tear, I will obtain a magnetic resonance imaging (MRI) and consider operative treatment earlier if a large tear is demonstrated.

I obtain plain film radiographs of the shoulder on all patients. Common arthritides of the glenohumeral and acromioclavicular joints as well as calcific tendonitis should be excluded. Acromial morphology should be assessed by the supraspinatus outlet view, with the x-ray beam directed posterior to anterior in the plane of the scapula, but angled 10 degrees caudad. Acromial morphology has classically been described as being type I (flat), type II (curved), and type III (hooked). In their original clinical series of 200 patients, Morrison and Bigliani noted a high association of rotator cuff tears with increasing acromial morphology. Arthrogram-confirmed rotator cuff tear rates were 0%, 19.5%, and 88% in types I, II, and III, respectively.[2] Whether a hooked acromion is a causative factor or simply a concomitant finding in rotator cuff pathology is controversial. Regardless, caution is advised in diagnosing a patient with subacromial impingement in the setting of a type I acromion. MRI findings are usually nonspecific, however; they may include a subacromial fluid collection on the T2 coronal images, subdeltoid and bursal edema or fluid signal, with or without rotator cuff pathology.

I do not necessarily perform a subacromial injection in all patients, especially if it is their initial evaluation. Mild to moderate symptoms of limited duration can often be well managed with appropriate activity modification, nonsteroidal medications, cryotherapy, and, most importantly, an appropriate rotator cuff motion and strengthening program. Severe symptoms of protracted duration, or those refractory to the above-mentioned modalities, often warrant a subacromial injection.

In my hands, such an injection is both diagnostic and therapeutic. The most common therapeutic steroid agents utilized are methylprednisolone and triamcinolone, and are of equal corticosteroid potency. Most available studies have utilized anywhere from 40 to 80 mg per injection. I prefer using 3 cc of 1% lidocaine, 3 cc of 0.5% bupivacaine, and 2 cc of triamcinolone acetonide (40 mg/mL). The subacromial injection is made from a lateral site with a 22-gauge needle, directed toward the anterior subacromial space. The actual injection site is not as important as where you put the medicine. Anatomically, the subacromial bursa occupies the anterior one-half of the subacromial space. Needle length and patient habitus should be considered to ensure this target site is reached (Figure 2-1). After 5 to 10 minutes, I reexamine the patient and I ask them to quantify, in percent, their amount of pain relief when challenged with ROM and provocative maneuvers such as Neer's sign and Hawkin's sign. Initial failure to relieve 80% or more of the patient's pain should raise suspicion for another etiology. Although controversial, I believe that a favorable initial response to a subacromial injection accurately predicts the eventual clinical result after subacromial decompression.[3]

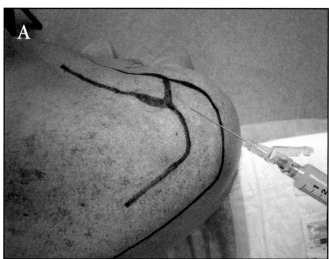

Figure 2-1. (A) Superior view. Patient's right shoulder landmarks demarcated (clavicle, AC joint, acromion, coracoid). Needle positioned superficially demonstrating planned posterolateral injection site and direction of needle towards the anterior half of the subacromial space. (B) Lateral view. Patient's right shoulder receiving posterolateral injection as planned. Dotted line represents anterior extent of subacromial bursa.

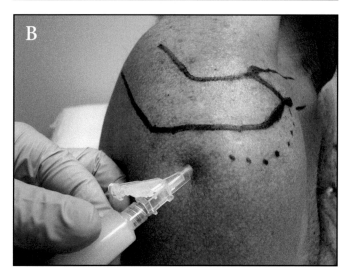

As is common in maladies of the shoulder, no single historical factor, physical finding, radiographic test, or diagnostic injection has been proven to be both highly sensitive and specific in the diagnosis of subacromial impingement. I prefer to use the constellation of clinical findings, including a good response to a subacromial injection, to make this diagnosis.

References

1. MacDonald PB, Clark P, Sutherland K. An analysis of the diagnostic accuracy of the Hawkins and Neer subacromial impingement signs. *J Shoulder Elbow Surg.* 2000;9:299-301.
2. Morrison DS, Bigliani LU. The clinical significance of variations of acromial morphology. *Orthop Trans.* 1986; 11:234.
3. Yamaguchi K, Flatow E. Arthroscopic evaluation and treatment of the rotator cuff. *Orthop Clin North Am.* 1995;26:643-659.

WHAT ARE THE PHYSICAL EXAMINATION FINDINGS (SIGNS AND SYMPTOMS, PERTINENT POSITIVES AND NEGATIVES) THAT DIRECT YOU TOWARD A DIAGNOSIS OF SUPERIOR LABRUM ANTERIOR TO POSTERIOR LESION?

Daniel J. Solomon, MD

Patients with superior labrum anterior to posterior (SLAP) lesions do not necessarily have a typical presentation, as there is often other shoulder pathology in addition to the SLAP tear, such as instability or rotator cuff tears, for which the symptoms predominate. Patients may, however, recall a specific injury with overhead lifting or a sudden forced abduction and flexion of the arm after which their symptoms began. Alternative presenting symptoms can be with proximal biceps tendon pain or vague anterior shoulder pain, especially during overhead lifting. Patients may experience a catching sensation or mechanical symptoms with the arm flexed and rotational torque placed on the arm.

Conditions in which the humeral head shifts superiorly, such as rotator cuff tears or the throwers' shoulder, may predispose patients to attritional tears of the superior labrum. Incidence of SLAP tears found during routine shoulder arthroscopy is between 6% and 12%, but is largely population dependent. Kim and colleagues found 26% of over 500 shoulder arthroscopies to have a SLAP tear, but 74% of those tears were type I tears.[1] Because of the high prevalence and overlap with other conditions, diagnosis based on physical examination can be challenging. High clinical suspicion, combined with specific provocative testing and appropriate imaging, usually leads to the correct diagnosis.

Figure 3-1. O'Brien's Active Compression Test is demonstrated. The patient's arm is forward flexed to 90 degrees and adducted to 15 degrees. The patient resists the examiner's downward force first with the arm in maximal internal rotation, then in maximal external rotation or supination. Pain during the internal rotation portion described as deep inside the shoulder that improves during the external rotation examination is suggestive of a SLAP tear.

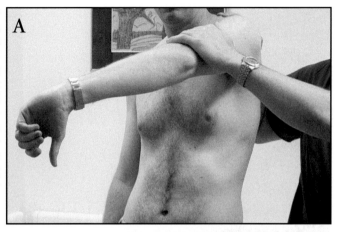

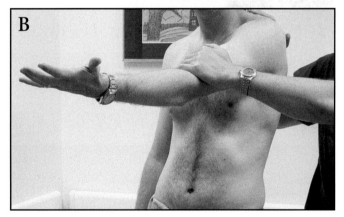

My preference for provocative tests for superior labral tears includes the Active Compression Test described by O'Brien and colleagues (Figure 3-1).[2]

O'Brien and colleagues found their test to be 100% sensitive, 98.5% specific, with a positive predictive value of 94.6% and a negative predictive value of 100% with regard to labral tears. Other investigators have not been able to reproduce their accuracy, but the test has proven quite effective.[1,3]

The Kim Biceps Load Test II is another excellent test that has proven quite useful clinically, though has not had as much scrutiny from other investigators as the active compression test.[4] Kim and colleagues found a sensitivity of 89.7%, a specificity of 96.9%, a positive predictive value of 92.1%, a negative predictive value of 95.5%, and excellent reproducibility with a kappa coefficient of 0.815 (Figure 3-2).

Given the prevalence of coexisting pathology, Speed, Yergason, apprehension, and Jobe relocation tests are all helpful, as are tests to evaluate the strength and integrity of the rotator cuff. Hawkin's and Neer's impingement tests are useful as well. Parentis and colleagues found no single test for diagnosis of SLAP lesions to be both sensitive and specific.[3]

Clinical suspicion must therefore be combined with a thorough shoulder examination and appropriate imaging with magnetic resonance imaging (MRI) or MRI arthrogram, for accurate preoperative diagnosis.

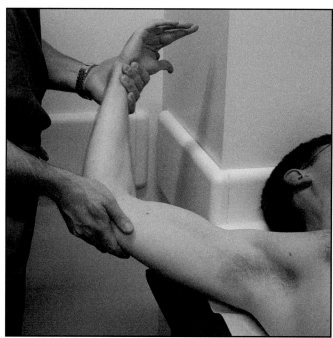

Figure 3-2. The Kim Biceps Load Test II is shown. The arm is elevated to 120 degrees. The elbow is flexed to 90 degrees and the shoulder maximally externally rotated with the forearm supinated. The patient attempts to flex the elbow while the examiner resists his motion. If pain accompanies his attempted elbow flexion, the examination suggests a SLAP tear.

References

1. Kim TK, Queale WS, Cosgarea AJ, McFarland EC. Clinical features of the different types of SLAP lesions. *J Bone Joint Surg*. 2003;85A:66-71.
2. O'Brien SJ, Pagnani MJ, Fealy S, McGlynn SR, Wilson JR. The active compression test: a new and effective test for diagnosing labral tears and acromioclavicular joint abnormality. *Am J Sports Med*. 1998;26:610-614.
3. Parentis MA, Glousman RE, Mohr KS, Yocum LA. An evaluation of the provocative tests for superior labral anterior posterior lesions. *Am J Sports Med*. 2006;34:265-268.
4. Kim S, Ha K, Ahn J, Kim S, Choi H. Biceps load test II: a clinical test for SLAP lesions of the shoulder. *Arthroscopy*. 2001;17:160-164.

SECTION II

IMAGING QUESTIONS

A 19-Year-Old Male Has Suffered Four Recurrent Dislocations During Sporting Activity. He Has Been Able to Self-Reduce the Last Two Episodes. What Is the Advanced Imaging Study of Choice?

Justin W. Chandler, MD
Alex Creighton, MD

When evaluating a patient with recurrent instability of the shoulder, we think that radiographic evaluation remains a very important part of the work-up. We always obtain standard radiographs including anteroposterior, axillary lateral, scapular "Y," West Point view, Garth view, and Stryker notch view to give important information about large humeral head and glenoid bony defects and their relationship to surrounding bony structures. However, in the case of recurrent instability, further cross sectional imaging is imperative for complete evaluation. Computed tomography (CT), CT arthrogram (CTA), magnetic resonance imaging (MRI), and MRI arthrogram have been used to further delineate intra-articular derangement in this setting. MRI arthrogram is clearly the imaging modality of choice in evaluating a young patient with recurrent glenohumeral instability.

We are increasingly using the advanced imaging techniques of CT and CTA because they have been advocated in their use for evaluation of bony insufficiency of the glenoid. Traditionally thought to be a rare cause of recurrent instability, a recent study found an osseous Bankart lesion in 50% of shoulders with recurrent anterior glenohumeral instability using three-dimensionally reconstructed CT images.[1] This is very important

Figure 4-1. A 14-year-old male suffered a shoulder dislocation, but also tore his subscapularis.

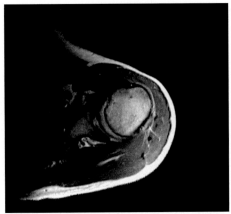

in surgical planning, as erosion or compression fracture of >25% of the gleniod surface was found to be significantly associated with failure of arthroscopic Bankart repair.[2] Another recent study using CT to evaluate glenoid morphology found flattening of the anterior glenoid curvature in 91% of dislocated shoulders, compared to only 4% in normal shoulders. The degree of flattening of the anterior glenoid curvature tended to increase exponentially with the number of anterior dislocations.[3] This study, however, found that three-dimensional reconstructions were not helpful and were of poor or noninterpretable quality in 41% of shoulders.

Although CT has been shown to be helpful for quantification of bone loss, it is inadequate for evaluating soft-tissue injuries associated with recurrent instability. We use MRI frequently to detect bone involvement and it is much better for delineating intra-articular anatomy and pathology. The addition of contrast greatly improved sensitivity and specificity of diagnosis of soft-tissue injury[4] (Figure 4-1). Chandnani and colleagues[5] found detached labrum were detected in 46% on MRI, 96% on MRI arthrogram, and 52% by CTA. Sano and colleagues[6] found 87% sensitivity in detection of torn labrum by MRI arthrogram, compared to 33% with CTA. MRI is also useful in identifying other lesions associated with instability including humeral avulsion of the glenohumeral ligament (HAGL), glenolabral articular disruption (GLAD), anterior labroligamentous periosteal sleeve avulsion (ALPSA), and superior labrum anterior to posterior (SLAP) lesions. Additionally, there is no exposure to ionizing radiation, as with CT scans.

We also consider the benefits of intra-articular contrast with MRI (MRI arthrogram). An MRI arthrogram allows gadolinium contrast injected into the joint to cause distension and allows structures to separate, providing a contrast of the structures within the joint. The drawback is that it becomes an invasive procedure, although it is well tolerated. MRI arthrogram is typically performed by injecting approximately 12 to 15 mL of gadolinium diluted 1:200 with normal saline. The solution is usually introduced through the rotator interval using fluoroscopic guidance with a 22-gauge spinal needle. Imaging should be performed within 30 minutes to minimize excessive resorption of intra-articular gadolinium. Protocols vary by institution, but a standard set of sequences includes spin-echo T1-weighted images with frequency selective fat saturation in the axial, sagittal, and coronal planes. At least one T2-weighted sequence is usually performed, which is helpful in evaluating rotator cuff tears, bone marrow edema, and paralabral cysts.[7] The addition

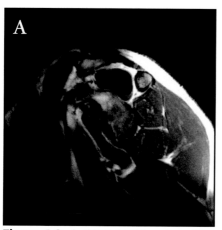 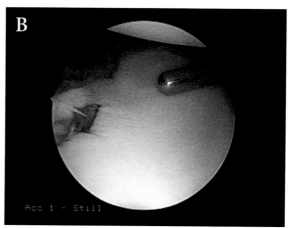

Figure 4-2. A 19-year-old male with recurrent dislocations and bony glenoid involvement. (A) MRI T2-parasagittal showing bony Bankart involvement. (B) Arthroscopic anterior view of "inverted pear."

of an abducted, externally rotated view has been shown to dramatically improve non-displaced anterior labral tears. This technique pulls the detached labrum away from the glenoid, allowing the defect to fill with contrast material.[8] Comparing conventional MRI to MRI arthrogram, Flannigan and colleagues[4] found that visualization of intra-articular surface anatomy was improved markedly after intra-articular contrast administration. They found that 6 of 9 labral abnormalities found with MRI arthrogram and verified at surgery were missed by conventional MRI.

Previous studies have shown MRI/MRI arthrogram to be inferior to CT for evaluation of bony deficiency[6]; however, because of the multiplanar capabilities of MRI, we have found that it can be used to adequately assess bone loss of the anterior inferior glenoid. En face views of the glenoid, such as in the sagittal oblique series, can be obtained and can provide a direct assessment of glenoid contour[3] (Figure 4-2).

When we are caring for a young patient with recurrent shoulder instability, the problem can often be more complicated than originally thought and may involve arthroscopic or open treatment with soft-tissue and bony reconstruction. Prior to surgery, it is imperative to have an accurate idea of the extent of bony and soft-tissue injury because this may dictate surgical treatment. MRI arthrogram is the imaging modality of choice—it will give you the most information about soft-tissue injury and in most cases will provide adequate information about bony deficiency.

References

1. Sugaya H, Moriishi J, Dohi M, Kon Y, Tsuchiya A. Glenoid rim morphology in recurrent anterior glenohumeral instability. *J Bone Joint Surg Am.* 2003;85A:878-884.
2. Boileau P, Villalba M, Hery JY, Balg F, Ahrens P, Neyton L. Risk factors for recurrence of shoulder instability after arthroscopic Bankart repair. *J Bone Joint Surg Am.* 2006;88:1755-1763.
3. Griffith JF, Antonio GE, Tong CW, Ming CK. Anterior shoulder dislocation: quantification of glenoid bone loss with CT. *AJR Am J Roentgenol.* 2003;180:1423-1430.
4. Flannigan B, Kursunoglu-Brahme S, Snyder S, Karzel R, Del Pizzo W, Resnick D. MR arthrography of the shoulder: comparison with conventional MR imaging. *AJR Am J Roentgenol.* 1990;155:829-832.

5. Chandnani VP, Yeager TD, DeBerardino T, et al. Glenoid labral tears: prospective evaluation with MRI imaging, MR arthrography, and CT arthrography. *AJR Am J Roentgenol.* 1993;161:1229-1235.

6. Sano H, Kato Y, Haga K, Iroi E, Tabata S. Magnetic resonance arthrography in the assessment of anterior instability of the shoulder: comparison with double-contrast computed tomography arthrography. *J Shoulder Elbow Surg.* 1996;5:280-285.

7. Sanders TG, Morrison WB, Miller MD. Imaging techniques for the evaluation of glenohumeral instability [review]. *Am J Sports Med.* 2000;28:414-434.

8. Cvitanic O, Tirman PFJ, Feller JF. Using abduction and external rotation of the shoulder to increase the sensitivity of MR arthrography in revealing tears of the anterior glenoid labrum. *Am J Roentgenol.* 1997;169:837-844.

WHAT ARE THE RADIOGRAPHIC VIEWS NECESSARY TO EVALUATE OSTEOARTHRITIS OF THE SHOULDER? ARE THESE ADEQUATE PRIOR TO TOTAL SHOULDER ARTHROPLASTY, OR IS AN ADVANCED IMAGING STUDY (COMPUTED TOMOGRAPHY SCAN, MAGNETIC RESONANCE IMAGING) INDICATED?

David L. Saxton, MD
Samer S. Hasan, MD, PhD

You can make the diagnosis of glenohumeral osteoarthritis and evaluate its severity with as few as two high-quality radiographs: a Grashey (true) anteroposterior (AP) and an axillary-lateral. The Grashey AP is obtained in the plane of the scapula and with the arm in 30 degrees of external rotation (Figure 5-1). This projection shows the glenohumeral joint space and the contour of the glenoid and the humeral head. The axillary-lateral view provides the orthogonal view needed to reconstruct the three-dimensional geometry of the glenohumeral joint. To obtain the axillary-lateral radiograph, the patient lies supine with the arm in some abduction and the x-ray beam is transmitted through the axilla toward a cassette placed over the superior aspect of the shoulder. A properly taken axillary-lateral radiograph will demonstrate the "eye" of the spinoglenoid notch and project the glenoid midway between the coracoid tip and the posterior angle of

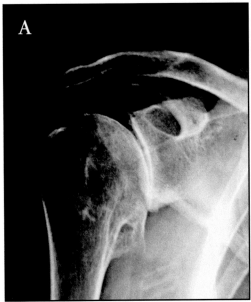

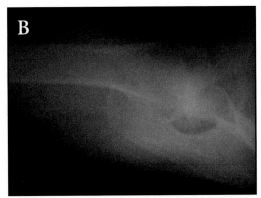

Figure 5-1. Representative Grashey AP (A) and axillary-lateral (B) radiographs from two patients with osteoarthritis. Both views demonstrate markedly narrowed joint space. Also note the "goat's beard" osteophyte visible on the Grashey AP radiograph and the spinoglenoid notch visible on the axillary-lateral radiograph.

the acromion[1] (see Figure 5-1). If the x-ray tube does not rotate or telescope adequately, an axillary-lateral radiograph can be obtained instead by having the patient sit leaning forward underneath the tube so that the beam is transmitted towards a cassette placed underneath the axilla between the abducted arm and the chest wall.

Both the Grashey AP and axillary-lateral radiographs demonstrate the characteristic features of osteoarthritis, such as joint space narrowing, subchondral sclerosis and cysts, and peripheral osteophytes. The Grashey AP demonstrates the osteophyte that typically rims the inferior humeral head, which Matsen and colleagues have termed the "goat's beard."[2] The axillary-lateral may demonstrate concentric joint space narrowing or posterior glenoid erosion and humeral subluxation.

When screening patients in the clinic, we often obtain three radiographs during the initial evaluation to help with the broadest range of diagnoses. Two of these are the Grashey AP and axillary-lateral, and the third radiograph is the scapular-Y view. The scapular-Y view shows the relationship between the proximal humerus and the "Y" created by the body of the scapula, the scapular spine, and the acromion. It also shows the contour of the undersurface of the coracoacromial arch. If we suspect on physical examination that the patient has symptomatic acromioclavicular (AC) joint arthritis, a fourth view is added—the Zanca view, angled perpendicular to the plane of the AC joint.

If significant cuff deficiency is suspected, with or without glenohumeral arthritis, then AP radiographs, with the arm in both external rotation and internal rotation, are obtained (Figure 5-2). The internal rotation radiograph enables an evaluation of acromion to tuberosity height. Gerber has shown that a height of 7 mm or less is a marker of rotator cuff irreparability,[3] or at the very least a marker of chronic and substantial rotator cuff insufficiency, which is helpful to know preoperatively. When imaging the shoulder with cuff tear arthropathy, AP radiographs reveal the amount of superior humeral migration from the center of joint rotation and the degree of instability of the center of rotation.[4] These are important factors in deciding preoperatively between prosthetic hemiarthroplasty and reverse ball and socket arthroplasty.

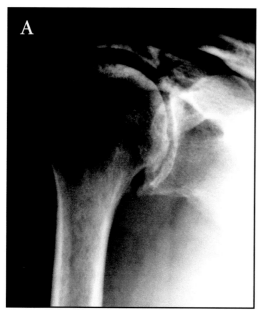 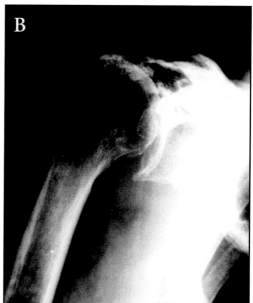

Figure 5-2. AP radiographs in external (A) and internal (B) rotation demonstrating decreased acromion to tuberosity height in this patient with cuff tear arthropathy. Also note the "femoral-ization" of the greater tuberosity and the "acetabularization" of the coracoacromial arch.

When shoulder replacement surgery is considered for osteoarthritis of the glenohu-meral joint that has failed conservative treatment, we prefer to obtain repeat radiographs within 3 to 6 months of surgery. A full-length AP radiograph of the entire humerus helps evaluate canal diameter and shaft geometry past the level of the tip of the implant when this level is not demonstrated on the AP of the shoulder. The addition of a scale rule to the AP radiograph of the entire humerus can aid in implant templating, but modularity and the prevalence of digital imaging have diminished this role. Full-length AP and lateral radiographs of the entire humerus should be obtained prior to revision shoulder replace-ment or when the arm has undergone prior reconstruction, such as total elbow replace-ment or internal fixation of the humerus.

In most cases of glenohumeral arthritis, the radiographs described above are adequate for careful preoperative planning. Gross rotator cuff competence can be determined and the extent of glenoid bone loss can be quantified as a percent of the articular surface. Significant glenoid erosion or biconcavity can be determined using the axillary-lateral radiograph. Obviously, a small rotator cuff tear cannot be ruled out by clinical examina-tion and plain radiographs alone, but if such a tear is encountered at surgery, it is usually reparable at the time of surgery and unlikely to influence outcome substantially.

The availability of advanced imaging studies makes it tempting to obtain computed tomography (CT) or magnetic resonance imaging (MRI) scans of the shoulder on every patient undergoing shoulder replacement surgery as part of a standardized preoperative work-up. However, additional imaging often adds little to the substantial information that can be derived from high-quality radiographs. In cases of primary osteoarthritis or nonerosive rheumatoid arthritis, when there is no substantial humeral or glenoid bony loss or deformity, radiographs are often all that is needed.

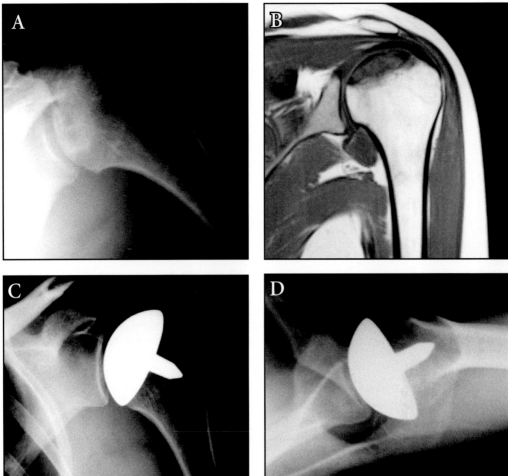

Figure 5-3. Preoperative AP radiograph (A) and corresponding coronal oblique MRI image (B) demonstrating osteonecrosis of the humeral head in a 30-year-old woman. The glenoid was uninvolved and the lesion spared the peripheral subchondral bone so that a bone-conserving resurfacing arthroplasty could be performed (C, D).

There are, however, situations when plain radiographs are inadequate or when additional imaging is helpful. For example, osteonecrosis may be suggested by patient history and plain radiographs, but MRI typically shows this more clearly and may help delineate the lesion so that less invasive options can be considered (Figure 5-3). MRI may also demonstrate glenohumeral osteoarthritis in its earliest stages when corresponding radiographs are unremarkable. Confirming the diagnosis of osteoarthritis helps direct treatment and patient education, even when shoulder replacement is not being considered.

Additional imaging is also helpful preoperatively in situations when radiographs reveal significant bony deformity or when high-quality radiographs cannot be obtained. For example, a good quality axillary-lateral radiograph may be difficult to obtain if shoulder abduction is severely restricted or painful. In certain cases of glenohumeral osteoarthritis, such as capsulorrhaphy arthritis arising many years after previous open nonanatomic repairs for instability, there is substantial posterior glenoid erosion (Figure 5-4). In certain cases of rheumatoid arthritis, the entire glenoid may be eroded medially.

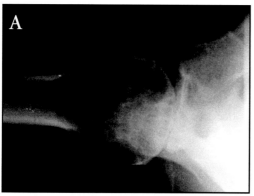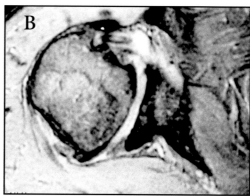

Figure 5-4. Axillary-lateral radiograph (A) and representative axial MR image (B) demonstrating posterior glenoid erosion in a 54-year-old man with osteoarthritis. The radiograph shows the humeral head articulating with the posterior glenoid and the MRI cut highlights the excessive glenoid retroversion.

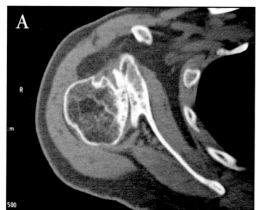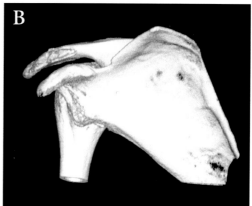

Figure 5-5. Representative axial CT slice (A) and three-dimensional reconstruction (B) demonstrating osteoarthritis in the setting of profound preexisting glenoid dysplasia. Identifying this degree of dysplasia is especially helpful when corresponding radiographs are difficult to interpret.

Humeral head deformity may result following proximal humerus fracture and subsequent malunion or following collapse from advanced osteonecrosis. In those instances, a more detailed preoperative knowledge of the three-dimensional bony anatomy is helpful, which can be provided by either CT scan or MRI. Also in our practice, patients often undergo an MRI evaluation of their shoulder prior to their initial presentation or request the study prior to considering surgery. When this occurs, patients are asked to bring copies of the images so that they can be reviewed preoperatively.

Because CT provides the greatest bony detail, it is the imaging of choice for cases involving severe glenoid erosion or dysplasia (Figure 5-5). Axial CT images can also be used to quantify glenoid retroversion more accurately and reproducibly than with radiographs.[5] It is true that glenoid version can be measured on the axillary-lateral radiograph by the angle subtended by the line joining the anterior and posterior glenoid edge and a line perpendicular to the axis of the scapular body, but the measurement is highly technique dependent.[6] One study demonstrated that glenoid version varied by up to 27 degrees depending on the angle of the x-ray beam and the rotation of the scapula.[6] Detailed axial imaging is essential for determining the potential for correcting glenoid version during surgery with asymmetrical reaming or bone graft augmentation. In addition, either CT or MRI can help determine if there is adequate bone stock to accept a glenoid implant.[7]

An MRI may also be helpful preoperatively when a substantial rotator cuff tear is suspected but radiographs fail to demonstrate fixed upward migration associated with chronic rotator cuff insufficiency, or the features of cuff tear arthropathy, such as a rounding off or "femoralization" of the humeral head and "acetabularization" of the coracoacromial arch shown in Figure 5-2. The presence of a large rotator cuff tear may impact surgical plan and prognosis because it may not be reparable and may tip the balance from total shoulder replacement towards hemiarthroplasty in order to avoid glenoid loosening from a "rocking horse" effect.[8]

When additional imaging is needed, we typically choose MRI over CT to avoid ionizing radiation and because of the added versatility of MRI in providing both adequate bone and soft-tissue detail for most situations. However, if bony detail is of paramount importance or if the patient cannot undergo an MRI because of intraocular metal debris, a pacemaker, severe claustrophobia, or another contraindication, then a CT of the shoulder without contrast is obtained. We specifically request a high-resolution study of the glenohumeral joint, as opposed to the entire shoulder or shoulder girdle, employing 2-mm slices with sagittal and coronal reformats. Three-dimensional reconstructions can also be used to "eyeball" the deformity (see Figure 5-5).

Summary

High-quality radiographs are the most important study for diagnosing osteoarthritis, especially in its more advanced stages. These radiographs are often all that is needed for preoperative planning. However, additional imaging studies such as MRI and CT are helpful for preoperative planning in cases involving significant glenohumeral bony deformity or rotator cuff insufficiency.

References

1. Matsen FA III, Lippitt SB. Principles of glenohumeral radiology. In: *Shoulder Surgery: Principles and Procedures*. Philadelphia: Elsevier; 2004:6-12.
2. Matsen FA III, Lippitt SB, Sidles JA, Harryman DT II. *Practical Evaluation and Management of the Shoulder*. Philadelphia: WB Saunders; 1994.
3. Gerber C. Massive rotator cuff tears. In: Iannotti JP Williams GR Jr, eds. *Disorders of the Shoulder: Diagnosis and Management*. Baltimore: Lippincott Williams and Wilkins; 1999:58.
4. Visotsky JL, Basamania C, Seebauer L, Rockwood CA, Jensen KL. Cuff tear arthropathy: pathogenesis, classification, and algorithm for treatment. *J Bone Joint Surg Am*. 2004;86A(Suppl 2):35-40.
5. Friedman RJ, Hawthorne KB, Genez BM. The use of computerized tomography in the measurement of glenoid version. *J Bone Joint Surg Am*. 1992;74:1032-1037.
6. Jensen, KL, Rockwood CA. X-ray evaluation of shoulder problems. In: Rockwood CA Jr, Matsen FA III, eds. *The Shoulder*. 3rd ed. Philadelphia: WB Saunders; 2004:187-222.
7. Kwon YW, Powell KA, Yum JK, Brems JJ, Iannotti JP. Use of three-dimensional computed tomography for the analysis of the glenoid anatomy. *J Shoulder Elbow Surg*. 2005;14:85-90.
8. Franklin JL, Barrett WP, Jackins SE, Matsen FA 3rd. Glenoid loosening in total shoulder arthroplasty. Association with rotator cuff deficiency. *J Arthroplasty*. 1988;3:39-46.

What Is the Imaging Modality to Best Diagnose a Superior Labrum Anterior to Posterior Tear and What Does It Look Like?

Craig S. Mauro, MD
Mark W. Rodosky, MD

We prefer to obtain a magnetic resonance arthrogram (MRI arthogram) with an intra-articular injection of gadolinium when a superior labrum anterior to posterior (SLAP) lesion is suspected. Although we feel that MR anthrography is the most sensitive modality to determine a SLAP tear, conventional magnetic resonance imaging (MRI) may also identify the lesion. In the Snyder classification of SLAP lesions, type I is defined as superior labral fraying with an intact attachment of the biceps tendon. Type II is defined as tearing with detachment of the biceps anchor from the supraglenoid tubercle. Type III is defined as a bucket-handle displacement of the superior labrum with an intact biceps anchor, whereas type IV is defined as a bucket-handle fragment with the tear extending into the biceps tendon.

When we evaluate an MRI arthrogram in a patient with a suspected SLAP tear, it is important to remember that the superior labrum has an irregular shape and is hyperintense. The biceps anchor, however, appears stable. In a type II SLAP lesion, a line of high-intensity signal runs across the base of the hyperintense labrum to the periphery. The long head of the biceps tendon has normal signal and shape and is attached to the avulsed labrum. We also utilize MRI to detect supraglenoid cysts, which may be associated with type II SLAP lesions (Figure 6-1). There are also several types of findings on MR that we utilize to try to classify the tear preoperatively. With type III SLAP lesions, an undisplaced bucket-handle tear may be identified as a line of high-intensity signal coursing across the base of the hyperintense labrum. A displaced flap may be identified as a discrete piece of fibrocartilage within the joint capsule, whereas the biceps tendon

Figure 6-1. Coronal oblique T2-weighted MR arthrogram demonstrating a type II SLAP tear with a paralabral cyst that is multiseptated and extends to the spinoglenoid notch.

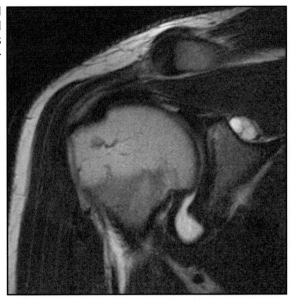

is attached to the supraglenoid tubercle. With type IV SLAP lesions, the superior labrum has a similar appearance to type III lesions. However, there is also hyperintensity and splitting of the fibers of the biceps tendon. Connell and colleagues correlated the findings on conventional MRI with arthroscopic surgical findings.[1] They found conventional MRI had a sensitivity of 98.0%, a specificity of 89.5%, and an accuracy of 95.7% for detection of SLAP lesions. However, other series have reported lower sensitivities and accuracies with conventional MRI for the detection of SLAP lesions.[2]

Normal labral variants must be understood because a congenital cleft and congenital variations of the anterosuperior labrum (such as a sublabral hole or Buford complex) can be misleading on conventional MRI. High signal intensity between the labrum and the glenoid in the posterior third of the superior glenoid is indicative of SLAP tear, as the superior recess does not extend posterior to the insertion of the long head of the biceps tendon. Secondly, a highly specific sign for a SLAP tear is two high-signal intensity lines in the superior labrum. Only one of the lines can represent the superior recess, whereas the other represents a SLAP tear. Finally, because the recess curves smoothly and medially as it extends over the superior glenoid, any irregular or laterally curved area of high signal intensity may represent a SLAP tear.

Compared to conventional MRI technique, we feel that MR anthrography with an intra-articular injection of gadolinium provides improved visualization of labral lesions. SLAP lesions may be appreciated on the coronal oblique sequence as a deep cleft between the superior labrum and the glenoid that extends well around and below the biceps anchor. Contrast may diffuse into the labral fragment, causing it to appear ragged or indistinct (Figures 6-2 and 6-3). The axial view is sometimes helpful to visualize the displaced superior labral fragment. Most series report the accuracy to be around 90% for MR arthrography in the diagnosis of SLAP lesions.[2,3]

In our practice, MR arthrography is ordered on all patients suspected of having a SLAP lesion. MR arthrography may be especially valuable and may yield more diagnostic information in the athletic population than conventional MRI.[3]

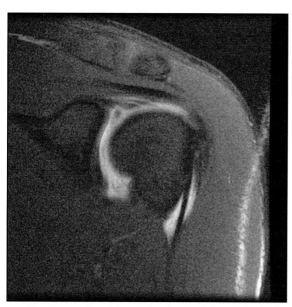

Figure 6-2. Fat-suppressed coronal oblique T1-weighted MR arthrogram demonstrating detachment of the superior labrum, consistent with a type II SLAP tear.

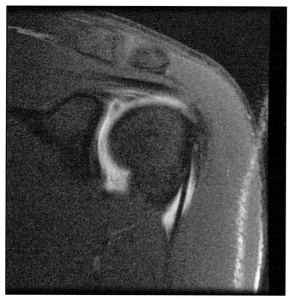

Figure 6-3. Fat suppressed coronal oblique T1-weighted MR arthrogram demonstrating a type IV SLAP tear with extension through the biceps tendon.

References

1. Connell DA, Potter HG, Wickiewicz TL, Altchek DW, Warren RF. Noncontrast magnetic resonance imaging of superior labral lesions. 102 cases confirmed at arthroscopic surgery. *Am J Sports Med.* 1999;27:208-213.
2. Waldt S, Burkart A, Lange P, Imhoff AB, Rummeny EJ, Woertler K. Diagnostic performance of MR arthrography in the assessment of superior labral anteroposterior lesions of the shoulder. *AJR Am J Roentgenol.* 2004;182:1271-1278.
3. Magee T, Williams D, Mani N. Shoulder MR arthrography: which patient group benefits most? *AJR Am J Roentgenol.* 2004;183:969-974.

SECTION III

SPORTS QUESTIONS

How Do You Manage the Long Head of Biceps Tendon in a 28-Year-Old Weekend Athlete With a Type IV Superior Labrum Anterior to Posterior Lesion That Involves Tearing Into the Biceps and Affects at Least 25% of the Tendon Thickness?

Craig S. Mauro, MD
Mark W. Rodosky, MD

In the Snyder classification of superior labrum anterior to posterior (SLAP) lesions, a type IV SLAP lesion is defined as a bucket-handle fragment with the tear extending into the biceps tendon. In general, management of type IV SLAP lesions depends on the age and activity level of the patient, the percent of the labrum and biceps torn, and the condition of the remainder of the biceps tendon. Preoperatively, magnetic resonance arthrography (MRI arthogram) may be especially valuable when a SLAP lesion is suspected. Further, MRI arthogram may yield more diagnostic information in the athletic population than conventional magnetic resonance imaging (MRI). In a patient with a symptomatic type IV SLAP tear suspected or diagnosed on MRI, we recommend arthroscopic management.

Our preferred technique is to place the patient in the beach-chair position, although this technique can be performed in the lateral position as well. A standard posterior portal is established with the arm at the side. The arthroscope is placed in this portal to visualize the glenohumeral joint. An anterior portal is created in the interval just above

Figure 7-1. A type IV SLAP tear demonstrating a bucket-handle fragment of the superior labrum with the tear extending into the biceps tendon.

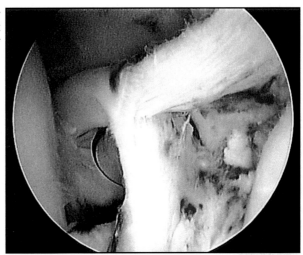

Figure 7-2. The extra-articular segment of the proximal biceps tendon is examined by placing a probe in the anterior portal and pulling the biceps tendon further into the glenohumeral joint.

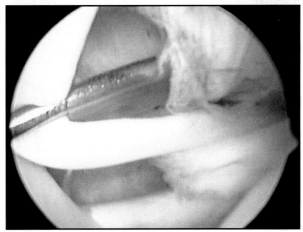

the superior glenohumeral ligament. After a diagnostic arthroscopy is completed, the SLAP tear is addressed. The tear is inspected to determine the extent of involvement of the labrum and the biceps tendon (Figure 7-1). The extra-articular segment of the proximal biceps tendon is examined for degeneration. This inspection is performed by placing a probe in the anterior portal and pulling the biceps tendon further into the glenohumeral joint (Figure 7-2). Further excursion may be obtained with the arm forward elevated and the elbow flexed.

In any patient population, when the tearing of the labrum and biceps involves less than 25% of the biceps, the torn portion of the labrum and biceps tendon is debrided. In this situation, the shaver is placed through the anterior cannula and used to remove the torn portion of the labrum and biceps tendon (Figure 7-3). In an older patient, or when the biceps tendon has significant tendinosis, a biceps tenodesis is effective. We prefer an all-arthroscopic technique called the percutaneous intra-articular transtendon (PITT) technique that can be performed with standard arthroscopic equipment, a spinal needle, and suture material.[1] However, a younger patient with a type IV SLAP involving at least 25% to 30% of the tendon thickness may benefit from repair (Figure 7-4).

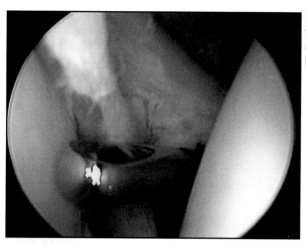

Figure 7-3. A shaver may be used through the anterior cannula to remove any torn portion of the labrum and biceps tendon.

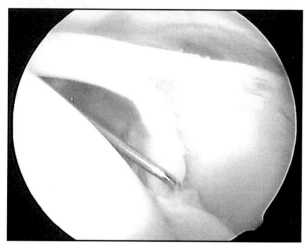

Figure 7-4. A type IV SLAP tear involving about 40% of the biceps tendon. Depending on the age and activity level of the patient, this patient may benefit from repair of this SLAP tear.

Our preferred technique for type IV SLAP repair is performed using a Spectrum (Linvatec, Largo, FL) suture-passing system to perform a side-to-side repair. To perform this repair, a Wilmington portal may be created 1 cm lateral to the junction of the middle and posterior thirds of the acromion, through the musculotendinous junction of the rotator cuff. The Wilmington portal allows a 45-degree angle of approach to the posterosuperior labrum and glenoid.

Postoperatively following a SLAP repair, patients are usually kept in a sling for 2 weeks. Active and passive range of motion exercises are initiated postoperatively, but strengthening is held for the first 8 weeks. Patients are released to full athletic participation or work after 6 months if all rehabilitation goals are met.

Reference

1. Sekiya LC, Elkousy HA, Rodosky MW. Arthroscopic biceps tenodesis using the percutaneous intra-articular transtendon technique. *Arthroscopy.* 2003;19:1137-1141.

A VOLLEYBALL HITTER HAS WEAKNESS OF EXTERNAL ROTATION AND VISIBLE ATROPHY OF THE INFRASPINATUS. WHAT ARE THE POTENTIAL CAUSES, WHAT ARE THE INDICATIONS FOR SUPRASCAPULAR NERVE DECOMPRESSION, AND WHAT IS THE OPERATIVE APPROACH?

Daniel J. Solomon, MD

When I evaluate a patient with shoulder weakness and visible atrophy of the infraspinatus, I commonly think about suprascapular nerve involvement. Compression of the suprascapular nerve in a patient with infraspinatus atrophy usually occurs at the infraspinatus fossa as the nerve courses around the base of the scapula. The nerve has already branched at this location and the sensory fibers for the subacromial bursa and supraspinatus motor fibers are unaffected. Ferretti and colleagues described suprascapular neuropathy in volleyball players in 1987.[1] Rather than affecting the supraspinatus and infraspinatus, the essential lesion in volleyball players affects the infraspinatus only because the pathologic condition affects only the terminal branches of the suprascapular nerve. In Ferretti's study, electromyography and Cybex testing revealed denervation of the infraspinatus with 22% loss of external rotation despite the players being asymptomatic.

Patients may describe vague posterolateral shoulder pain and decreased range of motion, specifically with abduction. The typical examination findings include atrophy of the infraspinatus (Figure 8-1) and weakness with abduction or external rotation.

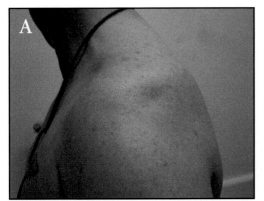 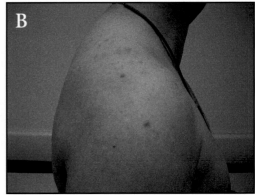

Figure 8-1. Though not a volleyball player, this patient has atrophy affecting the left infraspinatus from a suprascapular nerve injury. (A) Affected shoulder. (B) Normal shoulder.

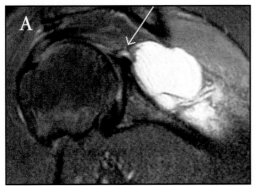 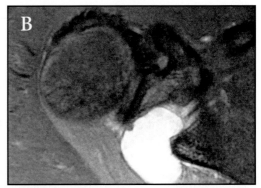

Figure 8-2. MR images demonstrating paralabral cyst in the spinoglenoid notch. (A) Coronal image; SLAP tear is also seen. (B) Axial image. (C) Sagittal image.

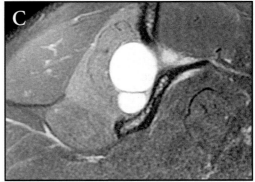

It is important to take a thorough history of prior sports and shoulder demands. The nature of the volleyball serve with infraspinatus required for braking the arm likely causes compression of the nerve. Spinoglenoid ligament compression on the suprascapular nerve is another potential cause. The most surgically treatable etiology is a cyst in the fossa adjacent to the nerve, usually from the glenohumeral joint via a superior labrum anterior to posterior (SLAP) tear and "one-way valve" effect. The cyst can compress the nerve, leading to weakness and atrophy of the infraspinatus in addition to the possible symptoms from the SLAP tear (Figure 8-2).

The differential diagnosis includes cervical disk disease, Parsonage-Turner Syndrome, rotator cuff tear or tendonitis, glenohumeral degenerative changes, posterior shoulder instability, and quadrilateral space syndrome.

I include standard radiographs to help determine calcification of the spinoglenoid ligament and magnetic resonance imaging (MRI) to evaluate the area surrounding the suprascapular nerve and muscle quality of the infraspinatus and supraspinatus. The SLAP region should be inspected carefully, regardless of presence of a cyst. Nerve conduction studies help differentiate the level of nerve compression as well.

My initial treatment includes rest and a directed physical therapy program for several months. Treatment directed at strengthening the teres minor and scapular stabilizers leads to the majority of symptomatic patients improving during that period.

If a cyst is identified on MRI or the patient has SLAP tear symptoms, surgical treatment should be considered if a period of therapy fails to curtail the patient's symptoms. Surgical treatment is more successful if the SLAP tear is treated in addition to decompression of the cyst.[2] A cyst compressing the suprascapular nerve visible on MRI and localized during glenohumeral arthroscopy with SLAP debridement and repair probably yields the most reliable relief of symptoms.

However, if the nerve is compressed by some other etiology, nonoperative treatment can be entertained for a much longer period of time and is often successful. If symptoms have been localized to a specific area of compression, I consider surgical decompression. Operative intervention for suprascapular nerve decompression can be performed via an open or arthroscopic approach. Open procedures for spinoglenoid compression involve a posterior approach. The trapezius can be elevated from the spine of the scapula, and the transverse scapular ligament is identified and divided medially. The suprascapular artery lies superior to the ligament and should be protected. By retracting or detaching a portion of the deltoid and elevating the infraspinatus from the inferior portion of the scapula spine, one can identify the spinoglenoid ligament and divide it laterally.[3]

Arthroscopic procedures should be practiced prior to performance and should be done by experienced arthroscopists, as the suprascapular fossa is unfamiliar territory even for experienced surgeons. Millett and colleagues[4] report on successful treatment of patients with paralabral cysts as well as those with compression from the spinoglenoid ligament via an arthroscopic approach. Rather than decompressing the cyst through the labral tear, Millett and colleagues recommend performing a capsulotomy at the posterior superior capsule above the labrum with the arthroscope placed in a transcuff portal for visualization. The supraspinatus muscle is retracted superiorly from the anterior portal. The cyst can be identified and resected with the shaver coming from the posterior portal. Additionally, the suprascapular nerve can be identified in the supraspinatus fossa and traced posteriorly to the spinoglenoid notch and decompressed along its course.[4]

References

1. Ferretti A, Cerullo G, Russo G. Suprascapular neuropathy in volleyball players. *J Bone Joint Surg.* 1987;69:260-263.
2. Hawkins RJ, Piatt BE, Fritz RC, Wolf E, Schickendantz M. Clinical evaluation and treatment of spinoglenoid notch ganglion cysts [abstract]. *J Shoulder Elbow Surg.* 1999;8:551.
3. Safran MR. Nerve injury about the shoulder in athletes, Part I. *Am J Sports Med.* 2004;32:803-818.
4. Millett PJ, Barton RS, Pacheco IH, Gobezie R. Suprascapular nerve entrapment: technique for arthroscopic release. *Tech Shoulder Elbow Surg.* 2006;7:89-94.

QUESTION

9

AFTER A "STINGER" DURING A FOOTBALL GAME, THERE IS WEAKNESS OF THE DELTOID, ROTATOR CUFF, AND BICEPS AND TRICEPS. WHY DID THIS HAPPEN AND WHEN WOULD YOU ALLOW HIM TO RETURN TO PLAY AGAIN?

Justin W. Chandler, MD
Alex Creighton, MD

"Stingers," also called "burners," are a common occurrence in all levels of American football, occurring in up to 65% of college players.[1] Also called transient brachial plexopathy, they are thought to be either traction or compression injuries to the brachial plexus or cervical nerve roots. Typically, the athlete presents with an inability to move the involved extremity and complaint of a burning sensation and numbness that is usually circumferential, rather than dermatomal.[2] The upper trunk of the brachial plexus (C5, C6) is most commonly involved and thus there is usually weakness in shoulder abduction, external rotation, and arm flexion.[3]

Three mechanisms of injury are described in the literature. The first is neck extension and ipsilateral lateral neck flexion, causing compression injury to the nerve roots due to narrowing of the intervertebral foramen. This narrowing is most pronounced at the C4/C5 and C5/C6 level, corresponding to the most common nerve roots involved.[4] Burners associated with this mechanism are more likely in more mature athletes with preexisting cervical degenerative changes. The second mechanism described is a stretch injury of the upper brachial plexus caused by lowering the ipsilateral shoulder and contralateral neck flexion. This is felt to be the predominant mechanism in younger athletes without preexisting cervical disease. Finally, least commonly described, is a direct blow to the brachial plexus at Erb's point, its most superficial location. This is located superior to the medial clavicle, just lateral to the sternocleidomastoid. A direct blow here can cause compression of the nerves against the bony scapula.[5]

Cervical stenosis has been studied as a risk factor using the Torg ratio of the width of the spinal canal divided by the width of the vertebral body. Meyer and colleagues found that college athletes with a Torg ratio of less than 0.8 had a 3-fold increase in sustaining burners.[1] Castro and colleagues found that the Torg ratio did not influence initial stinger occurrence, but noted that players who experienced multiple stingers had significantly smaller Torg ratios than those who only experienced a single stinger. They also noted that defensive backs were the most likely to experience stingers.[6]

Sideline evaluation of the patient should include a thorough examination of the cervical spine, including palpation for localized tenderness or deformity, and active range of motion within the limits of comfort should be checked. Thorough neurologic examination, including strength testing of all muscle groups, sensory testing in all dermatomes, and deep-tendon reflexes, is essential. The shoulder should be examined for injury to the clavicle, acromioclavicular, and glenohumeral joints. Symptoms may be elicited with percussion over Erb's point or with Spurling's maneuver. Any localized tenderness over the cervical spine or limited range of motion should prompt immediate cervical spine precautions and transfer to a hospital for radiologic evaluation to rule out cervical spine fractures, facet dislocations, or other cervical spine injuries. Stingers are always unilateral and any bilateral involvement or hemiparesis indicates a spinal cord injury and should be treated accordingly.

Management of stingers is largely supportive. Most resolve within minutes, without any residual weakness. The athlete should be removed from competition until all symptoms completely resolve. For a first-time stinger, the athlete may return to play the same day if the symptoms have completely resolved. Table 9-1 shows return-to-play criteria as described by Vaccaro and colleagues.[7] In 5% to 10% of cases, neurologic deficit may last hours, days, or even weeks.[5] In these cases, rehabilitation should focus on regaining strength in all affected muscle groups, and full cervical spine motion prior to considering return to play.

Prevention of stingers in football players is important and revolves around education, coaching, and equipment. Improper tackling techniques are felt to be responsible for many stinger injuries. Training to avoid head down tackling positions with knowledgeable coaches needs to be emphasized. Protective neck rolls and shoulder pads can be worn to limit cervical extension and lateral flexion and possibly decrease stinger injuries.

Table 9-1
Return-to-Play Criteria

No Contraindications to Return to Play	• Fewer than 3 episodes of a prior burner/stinger lasting <24 hours, with full range of cervical motion without any evidence of a neurologic deficit. • One episode of transient quadriparesis/quadriplegia with full range of cervical motion, no evidence of a residual neurologic deficit, and no evidence of a herniated disk or instability.
Relative Contraindications	• Prolonged symptomatic burner/stinger or transient quadriparesis lasting >24 hours. • Three or more previous episodes of either a stinger/burner or 2 episodes of transient quadriparesis/quadriplegia; the patient must have full cervical range of motion and strength without neck discomfort.
Absolute Contraindications	• More than 2 previous episodes of transient quadriparesis/quadriplegia. • Clinical history, physical examination findings, or imaging confirmation of cervical myelopathy/myelomalacia. • Continued cervical neck discomfort, decreased range of motion, or any evidence of a neurologic deficit from baseline after any cervical spine injury.

Adapted from Vaccaro AR, Watkins B, Albert TJ, Pfaff WL, Klein GR, Silber JS. Cervical spine injuries in athletes: current return-to-play criteria. *Orthopedics.* 2001;24:699-703.

References

1. Meyer SA, Schulte KR, Callaghan JJ, Albright JP, Powell JW, Crowley ET, el-Khoury GY. Cervical spinal stenosis and stingers in collegiate football players. *Am J Sports Med.* 1994;22:158-166.
2. Hershman EB. Brachial plexus injuries. *Clin Sports Med.* 1990;9:311-329.
3. Weinberg J, Rokito S, Silber JS. Etiology, treatment, and prevention of athletic "stingers." *Clin Sports Med.* 2003;22:493-500.
4. Yoo JU, Zou D, Edwards WT, Bayley J, Yuan HA. Effect of cervical spine motion on the neuroforaminal dimensions of human cervical spine. *Spine.* 1992;17:1131-1136.
5. Safran MR. Nerve injury about the shoulder in athletes, part 2: long thoracic nerve, spinal accessory nerve, burners/stingers, thoracic outlet syndrome. *Am J Sports Med.* 2004;32:1063-1076.
6. Castro FP Jr, Ricciardi J, Brunet ME, Busch MT, Whitecloud TS 3rd. Stingers, the Torg ratio, and the cervical spine. *Am J Sports Med.* 1997;25:603-608.
7. Vaccaro AR, Watkins B, Albert TJ, Pfaff WL, Klein GR, Silber JS. Cervical spine injuries in athletes: current return-to-play criteria. *Orthopedics.* 2001;24:699-703.

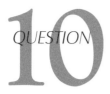

QUESTION

10

WHEN IS THE PATIENT ALLOWED TO RETURN TO CONTACT SPORTS AFTER AN ARTHROSCOPIC INSTABILITY REPAIR FOR RECURRENT ANTERIOR INSTABILITY?

K. Blair Sampson, MD
Samer S. Hasan, MD, PhD

Return to contact sports following arthroscopic anterior instability repair should not occur until the following requirements are met. First, the repair must successfully restore stability by clinical testing so that provocative tests such as apprehension, relocation, and load and shift tests are normal. Second, the repaired tissue must heal and mature and its biomechanical properties, including strength and compliance, must be enough to withstand the loading typically encountered during sports. Third, the rotator cuff and periscapular muscles must regain adequate strength, endurance, and coordination to maintain dynamic shoulder stability. Fourth, the athlete must be sufficiently conditioned and re-educated to play the sport properly and safely. Unfortunately, little is known about the time needed to achieve any or all of these goals.

Discussion about return to contact sports following arthroscopic anterior instability repair assumes that the repair is carried out properly. A poorly executed repair is more likely to fail than a well executed repair, no matter when that return to sport takes place. The arthroscopic repair must reattach the anteroinferior labrum tear (or Bankart lesion), which is usually present, onto the glenoid face to recreate the labrum bumper, and it must address any associated capsular stretch (Figure 10-1).

Refinements in technique have improved the results of arthroscopic anterior instability repairs. These include the use of suture anchors, trans-subscapularis portals for inferior anchor placement, posterior capsular plication, selective rotator interval repair, and surgery in the lateral decubitus position to enhance access to the anteroinferior quadrant. Careful patient selection to exclude those with significant glenoid and humeral bone loss has also improved results. The outcome and durability of arthroscopic anterior instability

Figure 10-1. Anterior labrum repair completed in the lateral decubitus position using 3 suture anchors and 2 posteroinferior capsular plication sutures.

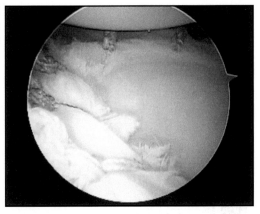

repairs are rapidly approaching those of the "gold standard" open repairs. Equivalently, arthroscopic repair is no longer contraindicated for well-selected contact and collision athletes with recurrent traumatic anterior instability and without significant glenoid or humeral bone loss. However, careful postoperative care, including compliance with immobilization, structured rehabilitation, and judicious return to sport remain essential to minimizing failure and optimizing outcome.

The answer frequently given for return to contact sports is around 6 months. Mazzocca and colleagues[1] retrospectively reviewed 13 contact athletes participating in football and hockey and 5 collision athletes who underwent arthroscopic repair. The mean duration for return to contact sports was 5.9 months and ranged from 4 to 10 months. Two repeat subluxations were reported at 22 and 60 months and required no operative treatment. Larrain and colleagues[2] reviewed the results of rugby players and divided them into an acute group of 40 patients undergoing surgery within 3 weeks of injury and a recurrent group of 158 patients. All players in the acute group had returned to sport at a mean of 5.3 months (range 4 to 7 months). Two repeat traumatic dislocations occurred at 1.5 and 2 years postoperatively. The recurrent group had 85% of patients return to play at a mean of 7.5 months postoperatively. Ten failures occurred, with 8 resulting from traumatic injuries during rugby and 1 each during tennis and polo. Postoperative time to failure was not reported and guidelines for return to play were not provided for either group. Cho and colleagues[3] reported the results of 14 collision athletes in a combined report on both collision and contact sports. The collision sports were judo, wrestling, ice hockey, football, and soccer. Three postoperative dislocations and 1 subluxation were reported. One of the 3 dislocations occurred 2 years postoperatively. Timing of the other recurrences and return to play guidelines were not provided. Although limited, the literature suggests a return to sport after 5 to 6 months, tailored to the individual patient.

Some data on return to play are also derived from the results of open stabilization, which differs from arthroscopic repairs in that the subscapularis is incised during glenoid exposure and its repair must be protected postoperatively. Pagnani and Dome[4] performed open repairs and allowed return to football after 4 months if manual muscle testing was equal to the other side. Out of 58 patients, none reported a postoperative dislocation and only 2 reported postoperative subluxations, both while playing football. However, no specific information was provided regarding mean times to return to play.

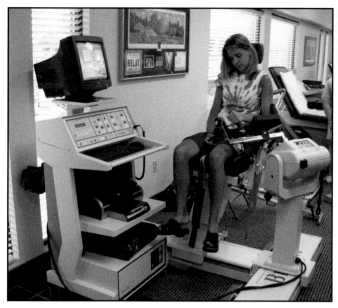

Figure 10-2. Biodex System 3 isokinetic testing system. The system can be used for both upper and lower extremity strength testing.

As arthroscopy avoids subscapularis injury, one would assume that returning to collision sports would be possible within the time frame for open repair, if not sooner.

The recommendations provided in the literature and suggested by the studies noted above are only loosely based on science. To our knowledge, no study has directly addressed the rates at which capsule or labrum heal to bone. Gerber and colleagues[5] reviewed the load to failure of infraspinatus rotator cuff repair in a goat model. Using a modified Mason-Allen type stitch through bone tunnels, the load to failure of the repair was 30% that of a normal goat tendon-bone construct at 6 weeks, 52% after 3 months, and 81% at 6 months. Obviously, human capsule and labrum may behave differently than goat rotator cuff, but the data reported by Gerber and colleagues provide an estimate about the rate of soft-tissue healing about the shoulder.

In contrast to the rough estimates about the time needed for capsule and labrum healing, recovery of rotator cuff strength and endurance can be evaluated objectively using isokinetic testing. Surprisingly, this technique is rarely reported in the literature. During isokinetic testing, internal and external rotation strength of the reconstructed shoulder is measured and compared with the opposite shoulder. Isokinetic testing, such as with the Biodex System 3 (Biodex Medical Systems Inc, Shirley, NY) (Figure 10-2), provides a reliable, quantitative method to evaluate strength, as well as an indirect method of gauging overall compliance with the postoperative rehabilitation program.

Our preference is to wait 6 months before returning an athlete to contact or collision sports after arthroscopic anterior stabilization. Athletes are cleared to resume sports without restrictions as long as isokinetic testing reveals strength within 10% to 15% of the opposite side (Figure 10-3). Football players are given the option of wearing a Sawa shoulder stabilizer brace (DJ Orthopaedics Inc, Vista, CA) or similar orthosis under their protective gear to limit shoulder range of motion as long as its use does not adversely affect their play. Athletes in other sports that permit bracing are also given this option, but athletes that participate in throwing or other repetitive overhead activity with their

Figure 10-3. Representative portion of a Biodex printout demonstrating bilateral shoulder internal and external rotation strength in a 17-year-old wide receiver 6 months following arthroscopic anterior stabilization. The athlete demonstrated deficits of less than 10% and was cleared to participate without restrictions.

		EXT ROTATION			INT ROTATION		
		60 DEG/SEC			60 DEG/SEC		
# OF REPS (60/60): 5		UNINVOLVED	INVOLVED	DEFICIT	UNINVOLVED	INVOLVED	DEFICIT
# OF REPS (180/180): 10		LEFT	RIGHT		LEFT	RIGHT	
PEAK TORQUE	FT-LBS	30.6	30.8	-0.6	53.0	51.2	3.3
PEAK TQ/BW	%	15.3	15.4		26.5	25.6	
MAX REP TOT WORK	FT-LBS	34.7	32.9	5.2	57.4	53.5	6.8
COEFF. OF VAR.	%	1.9	5.9		6.5	5.8	
AVG. POWER	WATTS	31.8	29.3	8.0	51.0	49.5	3.0
TOTAL WORK	FT-LBS	163.7	154.6	5.5	257.3	248.9	3.3
ACCELERATION TIME	MSEC	50.0	60.0		60.0	60.0	
DECELERATION TIME	MSEC	110.0	110.0		70.0	110.0	
ROM	DEG	76.1	75.6		76.1	75.6	
AVG PEAK TQ	FT-LBS	29.3	30.1		48.7	47.6	
AGON/ANTAG RATIO	%	57.9	60.2	G: 64.0			

reconstructed shoulder return to sport without any brace or orthosis. In certain situations, athletes willing to wear a brace during sports participation, and who have met all other conditions including isokinetic testing, are allowed to resume contact sports as early as 5 months. We remind our patients and their parents that the risk of recurrent injury cannot be eliminated, that trauma of sufficient energy will dislocate both normal and repaired shoulders, and that definitive return-to-play guidelines are lacking in the literature. Nevertheless, we feel this approach gives our contact and collision athletes the best opportunity for a safe return to play, and reduces the risk of recurrent instability of the repaired shoulder near to that of a previously uninjured shoulder.

References

1. Mazzocca AD, Brown FM Jr, Carreira DS, Hayden J, Romeo AA. Arthroscopic anterior shoulder stabilization of collision and contact athletes. *Am J Sports Med.* 2005;33:52-60.
2. Larrain MV, Montenegro HJ, Mauas DM, Collazo CC, Pavon F. Arthroscopic management of traumatic anterior shoulder instability in collision athletes: analysis of 204 cases with a 4- to 9-year follow-up and results with the suture anchor technique. *Arthroscopy.* 2006;22:1283-1289.
3. Cho NS, Hwang, JC, Rhee YG. Arthroscopic stabilization in anterior shoulder instability: collision athletes versus non-collision athletes. *Arthroscopy.* 2006;22:947-953.
4. Pagnani MJ, Dome DC. Surgical treatment of anterior shoulder instability in American football players. *J Bone Joint Surg Am.* 2002;84:711-715.
5. Gerber C, Schneeberger AG, Perren SM, Nyffeler RW. Experimental rotator cuff repair: a preliminary study. *J Bone Joint Surg Am.* 1999;81:1281-1290.

11

WHAT IS THE TREATMENT FOR A PATIENT WHO PRESENTS WITH A "SQUEAKING" SHOULDER 4 MONTHS AFTER AN ARTHROSCOPIC LABRAL REPAIR PERFORMED WITH A BIOABSORBABLE TACK?

Craig S. Mauro, MD
Mark W. Rodosky, MD

Any patient who presents with a "squeaking" sound following arthroscopic labral repair should be considered to have a glenohumeral loose body until proven otherwise. Work-up should consist of a magnetic resonance arthrogram (MRI arthrogram) to evaluate for the presence of a loose body, as bioabsorbable implants are difficult to visualize on computed tomography (CT) scan or plain radiographs.[1] Ultimately, however, the treatment for this patient is arthroscopy to evaluate the glenohumeral joint and remove any loose bodies before chondral injury progresses.

Sassmannshausen and colleagues described a series of 6 patients who underwent arthroscopic superior labrum anterior to posterior (SLAP) repair using bioabsorbable poly-l-lactic acid (PLLA) tacks (TissueTak; Arthrex, Naples, FL, or Bankart Tack; Bionx Implants, Blue Bell, PA).[2] The patients presented with persistent deep shoulder pain and mechanical symptoms at an average of 9.5 months postoperatively. Magnetic resonance imaging (MRI) demonstrated broken or dislodged tacks in all cases. Arthroscopy demonstrated unhealed SLAP lesions and broken tacks in all cases, articular cartilage damage in 2 cases, and no inflammatory response. Restabilization of the SLAP lesion with a bioabsorbable suture anchor was performed, and all patients reported improved symptoms.

Loose bodies may also be generated following rotator cuff or labral repair using bioabsorbable shoulder anchors. Barber described two cases in which bioabsorbable anchors used in arthroscopic shoulder surgery resulted in glenohumeral loose bodies.[3] In one case, a patient underwent an arthroscopic Bankart repair using Bio-SutureTak anchors (Arthrex) singly loaded with no. 2 FiberWire suture (Arthrex). At 6 months postoperatively, he presented with increasing discomfort with overhead activities and an audible "squeaking" in the shoulder. Although MRI demonstrated all suture anchors in their appropriate positions, repeat arthroscopy revealed a grade 4 chondral lesion with a 3-cm-long suture in the lesion on the posterior humeral head. The second case involved a patient who underwent arthroscopic rotator cuff repair with SpiraLok suture anchors (DePuy Mitek, Raynham, MA). At 6.5 months postoperatively, he noted the onset of sharp shoulder pain and, at 8.5 months postoperatively, MR arthrogram demonstrated a loose body in the shoulder. Repeat arthroscopy revealed part of the eyelet and upper screw threads of the suture anchor in the joint, but no articular cartilage damage. Both patients' symptoms resolved completely with removal of the loose bodies.

Bioabsorbable implants have several advantages over metal implants, including eventual reabsorption, improved postoperative imaging, and fewer problems with revision surgery. PLLA has become the polymer of choice for most bioabsorbable implants. Polyglycolic acid (PGA) tacks have also been used, but reports of early breakage and loosening, osteolysis, and foreign body reactions have led to concerns about their biocompatibility.[4] The rate of PLLA reabsorption is unknown, however, and these implants may still be evident years after implantation. In the reported cases of broken tacks, failure was observed in the shaft, just under the tack head. This area corresponds to the zone of transition between the portion imbedded in glenoid bone and the area that pierces the labrum. Further, inspection of broken PLLA tacks demonstrated no evidence of biodegradation.[2]

Bioabsorbable suture anchors may present a problem when combined with nonabsorbable sutures or those with slower degradation profiles. Also, complications may arise if the anchor is placed such that a portion of the anchor eyelet or the upper portion of the anchor is exposed. In this situation, the anchor eyelet may be subjected to cyclic stress as the bioabsorbable anchor reabsorbs. The anchor eyelet may have the potential to separate and become a loose body.[3] It is important to remember, however, that although repair failure can occur at the anchor, tendon, or suture, the weakest point of a repair is the suture tendon interface.

Surgeons who use these bioabsorbable implants must be aware of the potential complications. Careful surgical technique and appropriate postoperative rehabilitation are certainly the most important steps to prevent problems with bioabsorbable tacks or suture anchors. Inadequate burying of the tack or anchor eyelet, insecure placement of the device, or unobserved breakage during insertion may lead to problems. If a patient presents with a squeaking sound or persistent complaints postoperatively, an MRI arthrogram may help to diagnose the problem, but arthroscopy and loose body removal is the definitive management.

References

1. Major NM, Banks MC. MR imaging of complications of loose surgical tacks in the shoulder. *Am J Roentgenol.* 2003;180:377-380.
2. Sassmannshausen G, Sukay M, Mair SD. Broken or dislodged poly-L-lactic acid bioabsorbable tacks in patients after SLAP lesion surgery. *Arthroscopy.* 2006;22:615-619.
3. Barber FA. Biodegradable shoulder anchors have unique modes of failure. *Arthroscopy.* 2007;23:316-320.
4. Weiler A, Hoffmann RF, Stahelin AC, Helling HJ, Sudkamp NP. Biodegradable implants in sports medicine: the biological base. *Arthroscopy.* 2000;16:305-321.

SECTION IV

PEDIATRIC QUESTIONS

12

A 14-Year-Old Pitcher Presents With Shoulder and Arm Pain. It Is Midseason. There Is No Instability, and the Pain Is Primarily Over the Lateral Deltoid. Radiographs Reveal Widening of the Lateral Aspect of the Proximal Humeral Physis. What Is the Diagnosis and Treatment Strategy?

Christopher Dewing, MD
Matthew T. Provencher, MD, LCDR, MC, USNR

Initially described by Dotter[1] in 1953, Little Leaguer's shoulder has become the popular term for what is more accurately termed proximal humeral epiphysiolysis. Most agree that the injury can be attributed to physeal microtrauma in the adolescent athlete from repetitive hard throwing and pitching.[2] Due to the pyramidal shape of the proximal humeral physis and the thick overlying periosteum, displaced physeal stress fractures are rare.[3]

Teenaged throwers, most frequently baseball pitchers, usually complain of the insidious onset of pain at the lateral shoulder, radiating into the deltoid that worsens with throwing activity. We make the diagnosis primarily by history and physical examination, using radiographs for confirmation. The largest series of Little Leaguer's shoulder reported a mean age of 14 years and 83% of players were pitchers.[3] Most players reported several months of increasing pain with throwing activity, not restricted to any specific phase of the throwing cycle.[3] On physical examination, we usually find tenderness to palpation at the anterolateral aspect of the proximal shoulder. Occasionally weakness is present with resisted external rotation, but loss of motion is rare.[2] It should be noted that 80% of the overall longitudinal growth of the humerus comes from the proximal physis, and injuries to this area in growing adolescents may be problematic for limb length and deformity.[2]

We typically order the standard shoulder series with an additional anteroposterior (AP) view of the proximal humerus in external rotation, which reveals the lateral aspect of the physis.[2] In most cases, there is widening of the physis and often there is lateral metaphyseal fragmentation or sclerosis.[3] We have not found the need for advanced imaging studies.

Treatment consists of an initial period of rest and complete cessation of throwing activity. Carson and Gasser[3] showed a 91% return to sport after an average rest period of 3 months. There was only one premature physeal closure in their series, which did not impact limb length or function. We often counsel Little League pitchers and their parents and coaches that return to pitching should be delayed until the following preseason. In general, we begin gentle throwing drills once patients are pain-free on examination. If patients remain asymptomatic with throwing drills, we allow them to advance to hard throwing as tolerated. We advise players to adhere to current guidelines on age-dependent pitch counts and to work with their coaches on proper throwing mechanics.[4,5] Many Little League organizations throughout the country are adopting stricter guidelines on pitch counts, and several have outlawed the use of "junk" or curve-ball throwing. Current recommendations have been developed in conjunction with the American Sports Medicine Institute and can be found at www.littleleague.org/media/Pitch_Count_Publication.pdf.

References

1. Dotter WE. Little leaguer's shoulder. *Guthrie Clin Bull.* 1953;23:68.
2. Chen FS, Diaz VA, Loebenberg M, Rosen JE. Shoulder and elbow injuries in the skeletally immature athlete. *J Am Acad Orthop Surg.* 2005;13:172-185.
3. Carson Jr WG, Gasser SI. Little Leaguer's shoulder. *Am J Sports Med.* 1998;26:575-580.
4. Lyman S, Fleisig GS, Andrews JR, Osinski ED. Effect of pitch type, pitch count and pitching mechanics on risk of elbow and shoulder pain in youth baseball pitchers. *Am J Sports Med.* 2002;30:463-468.
5. Kocher MS, Waters PM, Micheli LJ. Upper extremity injuries in the pediatric athlete. *Sports Med.* 2000;30:117-135.
6. Riccio AR. Mason DE. Little league shoulder: case report and literature review. *Delaware Med J.* 2004;76:11-14.

13

HOW DO YOU TREAT A 14-YEAR-OLD FEMALE WHO CAN VOLUNTARILY SUBLUX THE SHOULDER POSTERIORLY AND ANTERIORLY, AND HAS A SULCUS SIGN?

Ed Glenn, MD

The short answer to this question is nonoperative when there is no history of trauma or antecedent event. The key word in the question is *voluntarily*.

Hyperlaxity of a joint must be differentiated from instability. Hyperlaxity is increased translation of a joint with the absence of symptoms. Instability is a pathologic condition that results in discomfort to the patient. Generalized ligamentous hyperlaxity is commonly seen in the adolescent female population. The patient mentioned above has generalized or multidirectional shoulder hyperlaxity that is generated voluntarily by the patient. Gerber and Nyffeler[1] have classified multidirectional instability as a dynamic entity based on the presence or absence of hyperlaxity and based on whether the increased glenohumeral translation is voluntary or involuntary. In the absence of a voluntary component, multidirectional instability with or without hyperlaxity generally results from a single traumatic event or repetitive microtrauma to the glenohumeral joint. Voluntary subluxation of the shoulder in multiple directions is classified in a separate category. These patients report no prior traumatic event and often are able to reproducibly subluxate the shoulder at will due to asymmetric contraction of their shoulder girdle musculature.[2] Frequently, these patients will have some underlying psychiatric process or will voluntarily subluxate the shoulder for attention-gaining purposes. These patients should be treated conservatively with prolonged physical therapy and not offered surgical intervention.[3]

Evaluation should include a thorough history to elucidate any history of trauma or neurologic injury, previous shoulder surgery, or psychiatric history. Ask about any prior treatment for the condition. Physical examination should be carried out in a manner such that both shoulder girdles are completely exposed to allow full evaluation of the glenohumeral joint and scapula. Signs of generalized ligamentous laxity should be tested and include genu recurvatum, hypermobility of the metacarpophalangeal joints (>90 degrees of extension), hyperextension of the elbows, and the ability to force the thumb to the volar aspect of the forearm. Strength, range of motion, scapular dyskinesis, neurovascular exam, and glenohumeral joint stability in the anterior, posterior, and inferior directions should be carefully documented for both shoulders. Joint laxity is graded by the following scale: Grade 1+ (translation of the humeral head to the glenoid rim); grade 2+ (translation of the humeral head over the glenoid rim that spontaneously reduces when the translating force is removed); and grade 3+ (translation of the humeral head over the glenoid rim that remains dislocated when the translating force is removed). Radiographic evaluation of the shoulder should include anteroposterior (AP), scapular-Y, and axillary lateral views to rule out any osseous abnormality. In the nontraumatic setting (as in this case), some signs of generalized ligamentous laxity will be present, shoulder laxity testing will be almost identical from side to side, and plain radiographs will be normal. These patients will demonstrate no facial expressions of discomfort or will actually smile during the voluntary joint subluxation.

The mainstay of nontraumatic, generalized ligamentous hyperlaxity with a voluntary component is supervised physical therapy to strengthen the deltoid, rotator cuff, and scapular stabilizers. Patients and parents should both be informed early in the treatment course that surgical intervention is almost never warranted, and several months of physical therapy may be required. If the patient has an underlying psychiatric issue, the family should be referred to a psychiatrist for evaluation because the voluntary shoulder subluxation will not be eliminated until the underlying psychiatric problem has been identified and addressed appropriately.

References

1. Gerber C, Nyffeler RW. Classification of glenohumeral joint instability. *Clin Orthop.* 2002;400:65-76.
2. Matsen FA III, Titelman RM, Lippitt SB, Rockwood CA Jr, Wirth MA. Glenohumeral instability. In: Rockwood CA Jr, Matsen FA III, Wirth MA, Lippitt SB, eds. *The Shoulder.* Philadelphia, PA: Saunders; 2004:655-790.
3. Cordasco FA, Bigliani LU. Multidirectional instability: diagnosis and management. In: Iannotti JP, Williams GR, eds. *Disorders of the Shoulder: Diagnosis and Management.* Philadelphia, PA: Lippincott Williams and Wilkins; 1999:321-333.

SECTION V

TRAUMA QUESTIONS

14

A 16-YEAR-OLD HOCKEY PLAYER HAS A COLLISION WITH HIS ARM FORCIBLY EXTENDED. A MAGNETIC RESONANCE IMAGING SCAN REVEALS A LESSER TUBEROSITY FRACTURE WITH 2 TO 3 MM OF ELEVATION AND 2 MM OF MEDIAL DISPLACEMENT. IS THIS DUE TO THE APOPHYSIS OF THE LESSER TUBEROSITY? AND HOW DO YOU DIAGNOSE AND MANAGE TRAUMATIC FRACTURES OF THE LESSER TUBEROSITY OF THE HUMERUS?

G. Peter Maiers II, MD
Samer S. Hasan, MD, PhD

The 16-year-old hockey player most likely sustained a Salter Harris III fracture of the proximal humeral apophysis. The ossification centers of the humeral head, greater tuberosity, and lesser tuberosity appear at the time of birth, around age 3, and around age 5, respectively. These 3 growth centers coalesce between ages 5 and 7. The growth plate closes between ages 14 and 17 in females and ages 16 and 18 in males.[1]

Figure 14-1. Axillary-lateral radiograph demonstrating lesser tuberosity avulsion in a 15-year-old male who injured his shoulder playing football. Note the lesser tuberosity fragments (white arrow). Anteroposterior radiograph did not demonstrate the fracture (inset). (Courtesy of Nikhil N. Verma, MD, and Matthew L. Busam, MD.)

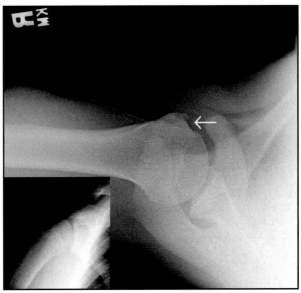

Because this injury is most commonly a result of significant shoulder trauma, it is important to first obtain a detailed history regarding the traumatic episode. It is also necessary to exclude concurrent injury, such as closed head or cervical spine injury. After the secondary survey has been performed, the focus returns to the injured extremity. Examination of the shoulder begins with careful inspection and includes an examination of the cervical spine. The affected shoulder is inspected for swelling and ecchymosis along the anterior aspect of the shoulder, often extending down along the medial aspect of the arm. Palpation of the anterior shoulder over the lesser tuberosity should elicit tenderness. Resisted internal rotation as well as passive external rotation should cause significant anterior shoulder pain. The belly-press and lift-off tests, used to evaluate subscapularis function,[2,3] are likely to be positive, but these may be compromised by pain.

Radiographic evaluation of shoulder trauma should include an anteroposterior (AP) view in the scapular plane and an axillary-lateral view to confirm that the humeral head is reduced (Figure 14-1). However, a lesser tuberosity fracture is often missed using these 2 views alone. If a lesser tuberosity fracture is suspected based on history and physical examination, then an AP view obtained with the arm in internal rotation may demonstrate the fragment inferior to the glenohumeral joint[4]. If a lesser tuberosity fracture is identified or remains in question, then a computed tomography (CT) scan or magnetic resonance imaging (MRI) should be performed to confirm the fracture, determine the amount of displacement, and help identify additional injuries (Figure 14-2). For example, Paschal and colleagues noted that the long head of the biceps is often dislocated medially in patients with lesser tuberosity fractures.[5]

Isolated lesser tuberosity fractures in both adolescents and adults are rare injuries, but 2 mechanisms of injury have been reported. The first is a forceful contraction of the subscapularis during resisted external rotation and abduction. The second is an axial load to the shoulder while the arm is extended and externally rotated. This mechanism may come into play during a fall backward on an outstretched hand. At the moment of impact, the humeral head translates suddenly and forcefully, increasing the tension in

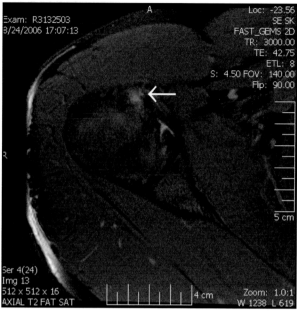

Figure 14-2. Axial T2 fat-saturated MR image obtained from the 15-year-old patient described in Figure 14-1. Note the increased signal at the insertion of the subscapularis, signifying site of lesser tuberosity avulsion (white arrow). (Courtesy of Nikhil N. Verma, MD, and Matthew L. Busam, MD.)

the subscapularis, the coracohumeral ligament, and the superior glenohumeral ligament, resulting in lesser tuberosity avulsion.[4]

In a patient such as this 16-year-old hockey player, who has a minimally displaced fracture with only 2 to 3 mm of elevation and 2 mm of medial displacement, we would recommend nonoperative treatment. We recommend a brief period of immobilization for 10 to 14 days, in a padded soft brace, followed by a structured physical therapy program. Sugalskie and colleagues reported on a 15-year-old pitcher who suffered an acute avulsion of the lesser tuberosity during the late cocking and acceleration phase of throwing.[6] The patient had a minimally displaced lesser tuberosity fracture and presented with pain and a "dead arm" feeling 19 weeks after the injury. He had been treated with rest, but had not participated in any physical therapy. A structured rehabilitation program that included rotator cuff strengthening, shoulder range of motion exercises, and a progressive throwing program was initiated. After 9 weeks of therapy, the patient was able to return to pitching at preinjury level. One year after the initiation of treatment, the patient was still pitching at the same level without pain.[6]

Radiographic indications for operative treatment include fracture displacement greater than 5 mm and angulation greater than 45 degrees. Clinical indications for acute fracture fixation also include a positive lift-off test, weakness in internal rotation and loss of internal rotation mobility. Indications for delayed fracture fixation are persistent pain and weakness despite strict adherence to the nonoperative treatment plan. When indicated, operative intervention in adults is through a deltopectoral approach and typically involves open reduction and internal fixation (ORIF) with small-fragment (3.5-mm) screws. If conservative treatment failed or if follow-up radiographs demonstrated further displacement, then we would perform open reduction and screw fixation in patients who are at or near skeletal maturity (such as the patient in the question). In a younger adolescent, we would be more concerned over the risk of iatrogenic injury to the physis. In addition to screw fixation, a combination of transosseous sutures and suture anchors can be used to repair the lesser tuberosity. Levine and colleagues described a technique using transosseous tunnels placed from the defect into the medial aspect of the intertubercular groove.[7] No. 2 Fiberwire sutures (Arthrex, Naples, FL) were used to secure the lesser tuberosity fragment and attached subscapularis to bone. Bioabsorbable suture anchors (Bio-Suture Tak; Arthrex, Naples, FL) were also placed in the defect so that the suture limbs could be passed through the subscapularis just medial to the lesser tuberosity apophysis.[7]

Ogawa and Takahashi reported excellent results with acute operative management of lesser tuberosity fractures in 2 of 3 patients, with satisfactory results in 1 patient.[4] They reported only satisfactory results with nonoperative treatment of 3 acute cases. However, all of these patients had displacement of more than 5 mm and angulation of at least 45 degrees. The authors also reported excellent results in 4 patients with chronic lesser tuberosity fractures.[4] Two patients were treated with nonunion takedown followed by ORIF and 2 patients were treated with physical therapy.

In summary, lesser tuberosity avulsion fractures are exceedingly rare injuries in adolescents, but they should be considered in the differential diagnosis of acute anterior shoulder pain following trauma. Displaced fractures benefit from early surgical intervention, but minimally or nondisplaced fractures appear to respond well to conservative treatment.

References

1. Webb LX, Mooney JF. Fractures and dislocations about the shoulder. In: Green NE, Swiontkowski MF 3rd, eds. *Fractures in Children.* Philadelphia: Elsevier; 2003:334.
2. Gerber C, Hersche O, Farron A. Isolated rupture of the subscapularis tendon: results of operative repair. *J Bone Joint Surg Am.* 1996;78:1015-1023.
3. Hertel R, Ballmer F, Lombert SM, Gerber C. Lag signs in the diagnosis of rotator cuff rupture. *J Shoulder Elbow Surg.* 1996;5:307-313.
4. Ogawa K, Takahashi M. Long-term outcome of isolated lesser tuberosity fractures of the humerus. *J Trauma.* 1996;42:955-959.
5. Paschal SO, Hutton KS, Weatherall PT. Isolated avulsion fracture of the lesser tuberosity of the humerus in adolescents. A report of two cases. *J Bone Joint Surg Am.* 1995;77:1427-1430.
6. Sugalski M, Hyman J, Ahmad C. Avulsion fracture of the lesser tuberosity in an adolescent baseball pitcher. A case report. *Am J Sports Med.* 2004:32:793-796.
7. Levine B, Pereira D, Rosen J. Avulsion fractures of the lesser tuberosity of the humerus in adolescents: review of the literature and case report. *J Orthop Trauma.* 2005;19:349-352.

15

WHAT ARE THE INDICATIONS FOR OPEN REDUCTION AND INTERNAL FIXATION OF AN ISOLATED GREATER TUBEROSITY FRACTURE, AND WHAT APPROACH AND OPERATIVE TECHNIQUE ARE APPROPRIATE?

R. Bryan Butler, MD
Anand Murthi, MD

When we take a history of a patient with an isolated greater tuberosity (GT) fracture, we find that the fracture usually has occurred by either impaction onto the shoulder or avulsion and shear mechanism. GT fractures can also occur with traumatic anterior shoulder dislocations. Displacement of such fractures can lead to shoulder dysfunction from decreased elevation and strength secondary to a loss of the supraspinatus moment arm with superior displacement of the tuberosity. With posterior displacement of the fragment, there is a rotator cuff tear and the external rotators will be lax. Furthermore, displacement of the tuberosity can cause impingement onto the acromion in abduction and onto the glenoid in external rotation, which can lead to pain and stiffness. The question then becomes, at what degree of displacement and by which technique should an isolated GT fracture be repaired to maximize function?

Although we have all been taught for years that the original Neer criteria[1] of greater than 1 cm of displacement and 45 degrees of angulation are a surgical indication for treatment, this may not be the case currently. Data are available to suggest that 5 mm of displacement is the criterion for reduction and fixation, with others proposing 3 mm in young, active patients.[2] Before treatment can begin, however, it is important to obtain adequate images because assessment of displacement will influence treatment. An anteroposterior (AP) view of the shoulder in external rotation or a true AP view best evaluates superior displacement, and an axillary-lateral view best evaluates posterior

Figure 15-1. Diagram of the heavy non-absorbable suture technique. (Reprinted with permission from Park MC, Murthi AM, Roth NS, Blaine TA, Levine WN, Bigliani LU. Two-part and 3-part fractures of the proximal humerus treated with suture fixation. *J Orthop Trauma.* 2003;17:319-325.)

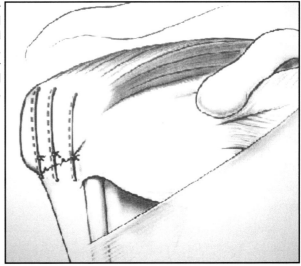

displacement.[3] Typically, we order a 5-view shoulder series for any new patient to assess fracture patterns, displacement, and glenoid involvement. Three atraumatic views of the shoulder (true AP, axillary, and lateral) can be obtained without having the injured patient rotate the shoulder into external and internal positions. Serial radiographs over 7 to 14 days may need to be obtained to evaluate for progressive displacement of the GT fragment. When evaluating superior displacement, we have found that if cephalad GT displacement is present above the level of the articular surface of the humeral head as seen on a true AP view radiograph, it correlates functionally with abduction weakness and bony impingement and should therefore be repaired.

When we are considering operative treatment, 2 types of surgical approaches generally can be used for open reduction—anterosuperior deltoid split or deltopectoral. We use the anterosuperior deltoid split approach centered over the fracture for isolated 2-part GT fractures. An incision along Langer's lines is made, extending from the lateral aspect of the acromion toward the lateral tip of the coracoid. The deltoid is split in the anterolateral raphe from a point 1 to 2 mm anterior to the acromioclavicular joint to no more than 4 cm distal to the anterolateral corner of the acromion to avoid injury to the axillary nerve. That approach allows excellent access to the fracture footprint with rotation of the humerus.

The 2 most common fixation options that we use include heavy nonabsorbable sutures, especially for elderly patients with osteoporotic bone, and cannulated screws, with either an open technique or a percutaneous technique depending on the amount of fragment mobilization that is needed. We use the suture technique in elderly patients with osteoporotic bone; 4 to 5 number 2 nonabsorbable polyester sutures are incorporated into the cuff tendons and are placed anteriorly, laterally, and posteriorly in the fragment and then passed through corresponding drill holes in the humerus (Figure 15-1). The GT is repaired to the proximal humerus in an anatomic position at or below the articular surface, with care being taken to avoid over-reduction. Park and colleagues[4] showed 89.3% excellent or satisfactory results with this technique; additional benefits include limited soft-tissue stripping and the avoidance of hardware complications.

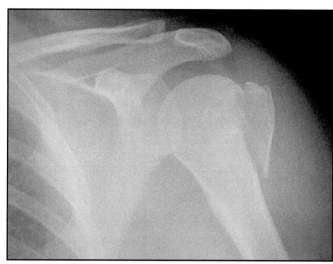

Figure 15-2. AP view radiograph of a 26-year-old right-hand-dominant female patient who was a pedestrian struck and subsequently dragged by a car. The patient sustained a left shoulder fracture dislocation. Radiograph obtained after closed reduction reveals a displaced, isolated GT fracture of the left shoulder.

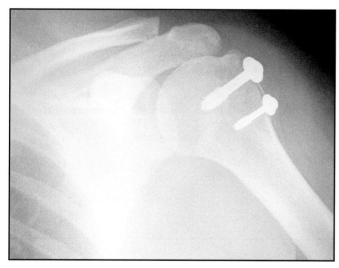

Figure 15-3. AP view radiograph obtained after the arthroscopically assisted, percutaneous GT repair with 2 partially threaded cannulated screws and washers.

Fixation with hardware, usually 1 to 2 4.0-mm cannulated screws, can also be performed. Percutaneous fixation with both percutaneous pins and cannulated screws has been described. Jaberg and colleagues[5] described a technique that uses 2 2.5-mm distally threaded pins inserted in a 45-degree direction through the GT, engaging the medial cortex of the humeral shaft. Problems associated with that technique, however, include pin infection and unexpected pin migration. Based on the same concept of the threaded pins, Kirshner wires (K-wires) can be used to gain and hold the reduction and 1 to 2 cannulated screws with washers can be placed over the wires to achieve final fixation. It is important to use washers if the size of the fragment is small or the quality of the bone is soft (Figures 15-2 and 15-3).

In addition to open and percutaneous techniques, arthroscopically assisted GT fixation has been described. The techniques combine the percutaneous technique of holding the fragment with K-wires and fixing the fracture with 1 to 2 cannulated screws plus using the arthroscope to visualize and hold the reduction with the use of the camera and graspers. Added benefits include intra-articular inspection of the shoulder to assess other injuries, such as rotator cuff or labral tears that can be associated with GT fractures, as is common with fracture-dislocations. This is a more difficult technique and requires experience in shoulder fracture management and shoulder arthroscopy. Last, for postoperative rehabilitation, the shoulder is immobilized in a sling for 2 weeks prior to beginning any formal therapy. A derotation wedge or pillow can be used with the sling to place the shoulder in neutral position. This can take the tension off the posterior rotator cuff and thus the fracture fragment repair. Pendulums can begin at 7 to 14 days. We follow the 3-step protocol of early passive range of motion for 4 weeks, active assisted motion and isometrics for the next 4 weeks, with no resistive strengthening until 8 weeks, as presented by Hughes and Neer.[6]

References

1. Neer CS II. Displaced proximal humeral fractures: part I: classification and evaluation. *J Bone Joint Surg Am.* 1970;52:1077-1089.
2. Park TS, Choi IY, Kim YH, Park MR, Shon JH, Kim SI. A new suggestion for the treatment of minimally displaced fractures of the greater tuberosity of the proximal humerus. *Bull Hosp Joint Dis.* 1997;56:171-176.
3. Parsons BO, Klepps SJ, Miller S, Bird J, Gladstone J, Flatow E. Reliability and reproducibility of radiographs of greater tuberosity displacement: a cadaveric study. *J Bone Joint Surg Am.* 2005;87:58-65.
4. Park MC, Murthi AM, Roth NS, Blaine TA, Levine WN, Bigliani LU. Two-part and three-part fractures of the proximal humerus treated with suture fixation. *J Orthop Trauma.* 2003;17:319-325.
5. Jaberg H, Warner JJ, Jakob RP. Percutaneous stabilization of unstable fractures of the humerus. *J Bone Joint Surg Am.* 1992;74:508-515.
6. Hughes M, Neer CS. Glenohumeral joint replacement and postoperative rehabilitation. *Phys Ther.* 1975;55:850-858.

WHAT ARE THE INDICATIONS FOR OPEN REDUCTION AND INTERNAL FIXATION OF AN ACUTE FRACTURE OF THE MIDSHAFT CLAVICLE?

R. Bryan Butler, MD
Anand Murthi, MD

Debate exists regarding the optimum management for displaced midshaft clavicle fractures. With evidence showing that union rates and functional outcomes with nonoperative treatment are not as high as once thought, operative intervention has become more prevalent in the treatment of displaced midshaft clavicle fractures.[1-3]

Zlowodzki and colleagues[4] conducted a meta-analysis of recent studies and revealed that the rate of nonunion for displaced midshaft clavicle fractures was 2.2% (10 of 460 patients) after plate fixation, compared with 15.1% (24 of 159 patients) after nonoperative care, a relative risk reduction for nonunion of 86%. Recently, the Canadian Orthopaedic Trauma Society[5] was the first to report results that looked prospectively, in a randomized controlled trial comparing operative plate fixation of 65 patients versus nonoperative treatment of 67 patients, for completely displaced midshaft clavicle fractures in patients between the ages of 16 and 60 years. The authors showed superior Constant scores and Disabilities of the Arm, Shoulder and Hand (DASH) scores in the operative group versus the nonoperative group. Furthermore, they showed statistically significant better nonunion rates in the operative (3.2%) versus the nonoperative (14.2%) group and better satisfaction with the appearance of the shoulder (83% versus 53%, respectively).

With all the recent literature on displaced clavicle fractures, the question remains: which fractures need fixation and which can be treated in a sling? Even though higher nonunion rates are associated with nonoperative treatment of displaced fractures, if one were to operate on all displaced fractures, one would be operating on patients who have a good likelihood to achieve satisfactory outcomes without surgery. The goal, then, is to identify those patients who would benefit from fixation by predicting those who would go on to symptomatic nonunion.

Figure 16-1. Radiograph of an 18-year-old right-hand-dominant male patient who was involved in a motor vehicle accident and sustained a shortened, segmental, displaced midshaft clavicle fracture with a butterfly fragment.

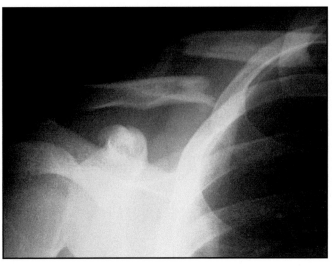

Most displaced clavicle fractures are sustained during simple falls, falls from height, direct blows, sports accidents, and traffic accidents. Fractures incurred during simple falls and falls from height occur more commonly in middle-aged and elderly persons, equally in male and female persons, whereas fractures in the young and predominantly male population are more commonly sustained during sports participation and traffic accidents. Furthermore, a large portion of displaced clavicle fracture incidence is incurred during motorcycle and mountain bike accidents.[2]

In our practice, absolute indications for operative intervention include open fractures, fractures associated with vascular or brachial plexus injuries, and fractures with skin tenting or compromise. Similarly, fracture shortening is one of the most well-known relative indications for operative intervention based on the objective criteria described by Hill and colleagues.[1] The study conducted by Hill and colleagues showed that fractures with *initial* shortening greater than 20 mm are more likely to result in nonunion, whereas those with *final* shortening greater than 20 mm are more likely to experience unsatisfactory functional results. We generally adhere to this indication and tend to operate on active patients with more than 2 cm of initial shortening.

Furthermore, another relative indication is the fracture of the middle third of the clavicle that shows a rotatory posterosuperior angular displacement of the medial fragment with a presumed soft-tissue interposition from the trapezius muscle preventing the fragment ends from contacting each other. Historically, such a fracture has been called the *irreducible clavicle fracture* and has necessitated operative treatment.[6]

Another indication to treat clavicle fractures operatively is the comminuted displaced fracture. More specifically, if a segmental butterfly fragment is present with significant displacement and shortening, in our experience, poor function secondary to medialization and ptosis of the shoulder girdle is likely to result, as are low union rates, and open reduction and internal fixation are required (Figures 16-1 and 16-2).

The method of fixation and the complications associated with operative intervention are important, yet variable. We prefer to use contoured plate fixation positioned on the anteroinferior aspect of the clavicle. We use plate benders and apply an intraoperative template on the anteroinferior clavicle. We contour the plate until it matches the reduction

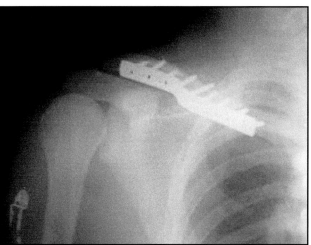

Figure 16-2. Radiograph of the patient whose image is shown in Figure 16-1, obtained after open reduction and internal fixation, shows a 3.5-mm limited-contact dynamic compression plate, which was intraoperatively contoured with plate benders, placed on the anteroinferior surface of the clavicle.

in both in the sagittal and coronal planes and rotation, which is key at the medial and lateral ends of the clavicle. Benefits to the anteroinferior position rather than the superior position include easier contouring of the plate, which is achieved by bending perpendicular to the plate rather than contouring in the plane of the plate. Also, in the anteroinferior position, less plate prominence is present and less irritation necessitating hardware removal occurs. We are careful to identify the supraclavicular nerve branches and to preserve them as much as possible during the approach.

Furthermore, we aim for at least 3 bicortical screws on each side of the fracture, preferably 4 for a total of 8 cortices, and frequently use interfragmentary screws for large segmental fragments. We routinely use a 3.5-mm limited-contact dynamic compression plate. Most fractures that require fixation are displaced rather than comminuted and have large segmental fragments or simple fracture patterns; thus they can be treated with compression and standard plating techniques. The issue with the Combi locking plate is that a longer plate is required to accommodate the number of screws needed for fixation, and a longer plate usually is not necessary in this patient population. Complications with plate fixation, regardless of the technique or the plate that is chosen, include painful hardware and local wound problems, which are issues that do not arise with conservative management.

Although no comparative studies have been presented, intramedullary fixation has been described as a treatment option for displaced fractures. Advantages include less soft-tissue disruption, smaller incisions, and less hardware irritation; however, nail migration, skin breakdown, and brachial plexus injury are real risks. I have had more experience with plating than with intramedullary fixation, and I think that plate fixation is overall safer with less serious complications. Hence, I tend to use plate fixation instead of intramedullary fixation.

Summary

I always repair a displaced midshaft clavicle fracture that is open, is associated with local vascular or neurological injuries, and presents with skin tenting or necrosis. Furthermore, fractures that initially are more than 2 cm shortened, that have posterosuperior rotation and angulation of the medial fragment, or that are large butterfly fragments with severe displacement also receive operative management.

References

1. Hill JM, McGuire MH, Crosby LA. Closed treatment of displaced middle-third fractures of the clavicle gives poor results. *J Bone Joint Surg Br.* 1997;79:537-539.
2. Robinson CM, Court-Brown CM, McQueen MM, Wakefield AE. Estimating the risk of nonunion following nonoperative treatment of a clavicular fracture. *J Bone Joint Surg Am.* 2004;86:1359-1365.
3. Nordqvist A, Petersson CJ, Redlund-Johnell I. Mid-clavicle fractures in adults: end result study after conservative treatment. *J Orthop Trauma.* 1998;12:572-576.
4. Zlowodzki M, Zelle BA, Cole PA, Jeray K, McKee MD; Evidence-Based Orthopaedic Trauma Working Group. Treatment of acute midshaft clavicle fractures: systemic review of 2144 fractures: on behalf of the Evidence-Based Orthopaedic Trauma Working Group. *J Orthop Trauma.* 2005;19:504-507.
5. Canadian Orthopaedic Trauma Society. Nonoperative treatment compared with plate fixation of displaced midshaft clavicular fractures: a multicenter, randomized clinical trial. *J Bone Joint Surg Am.* 2007;89:1-10.
6. Jablon M, Sutker A, Post M. Irreducible fracture of the middle third of the clavicle: report of a case. *J Bone Joint Surg Am.* 1979;61:296-298.

WHAT ARE THE INDICATIONS FOR OPEN REDUCTION AND INTERNAL FIXATION, AND INDICATIONS FOR HEMIARTHROPLASTY IN THE TREATMENT OF PROXIMAL HUMERUS FRACTURE?

James M. Paci, MD
Matthew G. Scuderi, MD

The treatment of proximal humerus fractures remains a significant challenge. The treating surgeon faces a number of important factors to consider preoperatively: fracture pattern, bone quality, fragment vascularity, as well as the age, medical comorbidities, and functional demands of the patient. The obvious goal of treatment is to restore a functional, pain-free shoulder, whether through nonoperative or operative means. The relationship of the tuberosities to the humeral head is critical to the outcome. On the other hand, the position of the proximal humerus relative to the shaft can tolerate moderate displacement in many cases, without compromising outcome. These important anatomic factors are often satisfactory with nonoperative management. When they are not, surgical intervention is warranted.

Minimally invasive, soft-tissue-sparing surgical techniques are preferable, but not always realistic. It is prudent to have more than one method of intervention available, in case any particular one is not satisfactory because of bone quality or comminution. For instance, humeral "head preservation" is often favored in most circumstances, but hemiarthroplasty should be available in the case that osteosynthesis cannot be adequately performed, particularly with more complex fracture patterns (ie, Neer 3- and 4-part fractures).

There are a number of options for "head preservation" when managing proximal humerus fractures, including percutaneous pinning, transosseous suturing, tension banding, intramedullary fixation, as well as plating. Regardless of technique, the goals of intervention remain the same: the creation of an anatomic, or near anatomic, stable construct while minimizing the risk of avascular necrosis. This can be a tall order, particularly in the elderly patient with osteoporotic bone. Therefore, each case should be carefully assessed on an individual basis.

The trend in the treatment of proximal humerus fractures has moved toward humeral head preservation. There are 2 major reasons for this: (1) the belief that secondary hemiarthroplasty after primary osteosynthesis has no worse outcome than primary hemiarthroplasty even if dealing with avascular necrosis (AVN) or malunion; and (2) the belief that "head preservation" surgery may provide better functional outcomes because the best contemporary studies show that <50% patients will be able to raise their arms overhead after hemiarthroplasty.[1] Furthermore, even in the case of head-splitting fractures, in a relatively young patient with good bone stock, open reduction and internal fixation (ORIF) should be attempted despite a relatively high rate of redisplacement.

Careful study of the injury films is critical. Films of the contralateral, uninjured side are often helpful for templating humeral height, version, and head size in the case that hemiarthroplasty is necessary. Close evaluation of the plain films can also be helpful in predicting the degree of periosteal stripping. An intact periosteum is helpful for closed reduction techniques, and perhaps more importantly, for maintenance of blood supply to the fracture fragments. When faced with a very complex fracture pattern a computed tomography (CT) scan with 3-dimensional reconstructions may be beneficial.[2]

Locking proximal humerus plates are quite versatile and can used for many fracture patterns. They provide more rigid fixation than convential plates, particularly in osteoporotic bone. Their anatomic shape permits better positioning, avoiding secondary impingement. Comminuted tuberosity fragments often cannot be fixed rigidly, necessitating the use of suture fixation through cuff and/or bone. The rotator cuff often provides an excellent source of fixation and should be used routinely. Even with open techniques, soft-tissue–friendly, indirect reduction techniques are important to maximize fragment vascularity and, hopefully, minimize the risk of AVN. In the case of severe metaphyseal comminution it may not be possible to reduce the articular fragment to its proper height. Minor shortening is often tolerated, but appropriate reduction of the tuberosities to the head construct remains critical to the ultimate outcome. The articular surface must be properly reduced for acceptable reduction of the tuberosities. Further, stable fixation with ORIF is important to permit early motion and avoid stiffness.

In the case that ORIF cannot be adequately performed, hemiarthroplasty remains a good option, and should be available as a back-up plan, particularly for complex fractures. The surgical goal of arthroplasty is essentially the same as ORIF: to restore the anatomic relationship between the humeral head component and the tuberosities. Preoperative templating, as mentioned, is very useful. Using the contralateral side as reference, if possible, seems to be the most reliable, especially for head size, humeral height, and version. Referencing the soft-tissue tension intraoperatively is often unpredictable. However, the pectoralis major tendon is usually unaffected by the fracture, and provides a consistent anatomic landmark. Its superior edge is typically 5.5 ± 0.5 cm from the superior edge of the humeral head.[3] Proper version is also critical to long-term success, but has significant variability amongst patients. As a general rule, proper version is restored when the head faces the glenoid with the arm in neutral rotation. Time spent on templating and planning implant position cannot be overemphasized. Early failures have clearly been associated with issues such as stem malrotation and head oversizing. Indications for immediate hemiarthroplasty are not hard-fast, but should be strongly considered in cases of severe comminution of articular surface, large articular segment impression fragment, or 3- or 4-part fracture in older individuals. Reverse total shoulder arthroplasty may provide an added option in some select cases, but its routine use cannot yet be advocated.[4]

Summary

Relatively simple nondisplaced or minimally displaced fractures are typically treated nonoperatively. Routine radiographic assessment is necessary to ensure maintenance of reduction. The use of the proximal humerus locked plate has become the primary treatment of choice for most displaced fractures of varying complexity. Simple suture fixation is sometimes used for isolated tuberosity fractures. ORIF is at least attempted for complex fractures and in patients with poor bone quality, but hemiarthroplasty is always premeditated in the case that an acceptable reduction cannot be obtained. It is important to emphasize that neither ORIF nor hemiarthroplasty are without potential complication. The recent report of the Mayo Clinic's experience with proximal humerus fractures noted a 51% early complication rate associated with osteosynthesis and a 64% early complication rate with hemiarthroplasty.[5] This highlights the inherent complexity of these fractures, and importance of careful attention to detail in each individual case.

References

1. Kralinger F, Schwaiger R, Wambacher M, et al. Outcome and primary hemiarthroplasty for fracture of the head of the humerus: a retrospective multicentre study of 167 patients. *J Bone Joint Surg Br*. 2004;86:217-219.
2. Shrader M, Sanchez-Sotelo J, Sperling J, Rowland C, Cofield R. Understanding proximal humerus fractures: image analysis, classification, and treatment. *J Shoulder Elbow Surg*. 2005;14:497-505.
3. Gerber A, Apreleva M, Warner JP. Hemiarthroplasty for proximal humerus fracture: a new method to obtain correct length. Presented at the 10th International Congress of Surgery of the Shoulder. Washington, DC, 2004.
4. Bufquin THA, Hubert L, Massin P. Reverse shoulder arthroplasty for the treatment of three- and four-part fractures of the proximal humerus in the elderly: a prospective review of 43 cases with a short-term follow-up. *J Bone Joint Surg Br*. 2007;89:516-520.
5. Smith A, Mardones R, Sperling J, Cofield R. Early complications of operatively treated proximal humerus fractures. *J Shoulder Elbow Surg*. 2007;16:14-24.

WHAT ARE THE INDICATIONS FOR SURGERY IN A SYMPTOMATIC SURGICAL NECK NONUNION, AND WHICH OPTION (OPEN REDUCTION AND INTERNAL FIXATION OR ARTHROPLASTY) WOULD YOU CHOOSE?

Joseph Y. Choi, MD, PhD
Matthew G. Scuderi, MD

Nonunion of fractures of the surgical neck of the humerus is relatively uncommon. It is seen after failed *nonoperative* treatment of 2-part surgical neck fractures and some 3- and 4-part fractures and often leads to significant pain and dysfunction. Nonoperative and operative treatment are challenging due to extensive bone resorption, severe humeral head cavitation, or glenohumeral arthritis.[1] Numerous approaches to the treatment of proximal humerus nonunions have been described, including intramedullary rods, tension banding, open reduction and internal fixation (ORIF), prosthetic replacement, and even intramedullary cortical bone grafting. In most situations, prosthetic replacement is reserved for older, sicker patients, introducing a significant selection bias when included in many reports.[2]

There are several studies that have reported favorable outcomes with ORIF for surgical neck fractures. In a retrospective study with 12-month minimum follow-up, 13 patients with 2-part nonunion of the surgical neck of the humerus treated with ORIF with bone graft were evaluated. Patients with avascular necrosis, post-traumatic arthritis, severe humeral head bone loss, or tuberosity nonunion were excluded. Isolated ORIF with autogenous bone graft yielded overall excellent outcomes, even in patients over 65 years old and patients with significant medical comorbidities. This treatment method offered predictable fracture healing with few complications.[2] In general, ORIF is applicable when there is good bone quality and the absence of significant glenohumeral joint damage.

Special care must be taken when addressing proximal humerus nonunion in the elderly patient. These patients often present with poor bone quality, severe resorption, and cavitation of the humeral head. All of these factors interfere with successful fracture healing.[1] In this group, arthroplasty may be an alternative. Twelve patients with surgical neck nonunions who underwent total or hemiarthroplasty were retrospectively reviewed with a mean postoperative follow-up of 69 months. Nearly 80% had complete pain relief and significant improvement in motion, which is similar to other published studies. Extensive releases, tuberosity preservation, and calcar grafting are important steps, especially in the management of these more complex patients.[3] In a subset of patients who have developed glenoid arthritis and rotoator cuff deficiency due to tuberosity failure after hemiarthroplasty for proximal humerus fractures, the reverse shoulder prosthesis offers a promising salvage-type of solution.[4] Reverse shoulder arthroplasty may also provide a reasonable option as an index procedure for surgical neck nonunions in carefully selected patients.

Summary

The decision to treat a nonunion of the surgical neck of the humerus operatively should be weighed carefully in terms of the risks and benefits to the patients. Although nonunion of the surgical neck is often associated with pain and severe restriction in function, nearly 50% of patients may be relatively asymptomatic, and observation may be warranted.[5] However, in a medically fit patient with good bone quality and the absence of significant glenohumeral joint degeneration, ORIF likely offers the best course of action. The alternative to ORIF is replacement arthroplasty; however, poor functional outcome remains a significant concern. Extensive releases, tuberosity preservation, and calcar grafting are critical to maximize functional results and pain relief.[3] In the setting of failed hemiarthroplasty, the reverse shoulder prosthesis seems to be a promising salvage procedure,[4] and may even be a viable index procedure for surgical neck nonunions in carefully selected patients. However, long-term results are lacking and this route should be taken with strict caution.

References

1. Antuna SA. Shoulder arthroplasty for proximal humeral nonunions. *J Shoulder Elbow Surg.* 2002;11:114-121.
2. Galatz LM, Williams GR, Fenlin JM,et al. Outcome of open reduction and internal fixation of surgical neck nonunions of the humerus. *J Orthop Trauma.* 2004;18:63-67.
3. Lin JS, Klepps S, Miller S, Cleeman E, Flatow E. Effectiveness of replacement arthroplasty with calcar grafting and avoidance of greater tuberosity osteotomy for the treatment of humeral surgical neck nonunions. *J Shoulder Elbow Surg.* 2006;15:12-18.
4. Levy J, Frankle M, Mighell M, Pupello D. The use of the reverse shoulder prosthesis for the treatment of failed hemiarthroplasty for proximal humeral fracture. *J Bone Joint Surg Am.* 2007;89:292-300.
5. Duralde XA, Flatow EL, Pollock RG, Nicholson GP, Self EB, Bigliani LU. Operative treatment of nonunions of the surgical neck of the humerus. *J Shoulder Elbow Surg.* 1996;5:169-180.

SECTION VI

RECONSTRUCTION
QUESTIONS

WHAT ARE THE INDICATIONS AND OPTIONS FOR GLENOID RESURFACING IN YOUNG PATIENTS WITH GLENOHUMERAL DEGENERATIVE JOINT DISEASE?

Joseph Y. Choi, MD, PhD
Matthew G. Scuderi, MD

Total shoulder arthroplasty has historically offered the most predictable functional outcomes and pain relief amongst patients with advanced osteoarthritis of the glenohumeral joint.[1] Unfortunately, in the active younger patient with glenohumeral arthritis, glenoid component loosening and polyethylene wear osteolysis are potentially devastating issues over the long term. As a result, alternatives to arthroplasty have been explored in this challenging population. Isolated humeral head resurfacing typically provides inferior results with regard to pain relief and function.[2] In addition, subsequent glenoid cartilage erosion is not uncommon, and may necessitate conversion to total shoulder arthroplasty.[3]

Biologic resurfacing of the glenoid in conjunction with humeral head replacement or glenoid biologic resurfacing alone for isolated glenoid arthritis is another alternative that may be appropriate in the younger population with glenohumeral osteoarthritis.[4] Biologic resurfacing avoids complications associated with prosthetic glenoid resurfacing such as polyethylene wear osteolysis, and glenoid component loosening. A variety of tissue implants have been tried, including both autograft and allograft.[1]

The best candidate is a young adult with severe bipolar (humerus and glenoid) degenerative disease with intolerable pain and compromised activities of daily living. Unipolar disease, or defects contained within either the humeral head or glenoid, may be amenable to focal cartilage restoration type procedures such as microfracture, osteochondral transfer, or autologous chondrocyte implantation. However, many of these techniques remain experimental or "off-label" in the shoulder, and are lacking long-term data. It is important, nonetheless, to define the extent of cartilage damage, so as to not "overtreat" the condition. Arthroscopic evaluation, with possible debridement and capsular release, often serves as a reasonable first step to quantify and qualify the status of the articular surfaces in those patients that have failed all nonoperative treatments. In general, it is felt that patients benefit most when intervention is early in the course of the disease with persistent joint concentricity and residual joint space.

A recent report assessed 2- to 15-year outcomes using humeral hemiarthroplasty and a variety of biologic glenoid surfaces.[2] Promising results were reported using American Shoulder and Elbow Surgeons (ASES) scores and Neer criteria, and favored the use of Achilles tendon allograft. Glenoid erosion averaged 7.2 mm and appeared to stabilize at 5 years.

Others have favored the use of lateral meniscal allograft for biologic resurfacing in hope to limit the progression of glenoid erosion and preserve bone stock for possible later conversion to total should arthroplasty.[1,5] Reported follow-up remains relatively short term, with promising outcomes in regard to pain, motion, and glenoid erosion. Long-term data are lacking, however. Static biomechanical studies demonstrated that lateral meniscus allograft interposition effectively reduces joint contact and pressure in cadaveric shoulders.[4]

Summary

Biologic resurfacing of the glenoid with humeral head hemiarthroplasty is a reasonable option for the treatment of end-stage bipolar arthritis in the active, relatively young patients with high functional demands, where total shoulder arthroplasty may not yet be appropriate. All other options for pain control including medical management, arthroscopic debridement, or focal treatment of unipolar lesions should be exhausted.[6] Patient selection and expectations are critical in the decision-making process. The optimal biologic resurfacing material remains somewhat uncertain. Major concerns with this technique remain, including deterioration of patient satisfaction, glenoid erosion, and the impact of conversion to a successful total shoulder arthroplasty.

References

1. Themistocleous GS, Zalavras CG, Zachos VC, Itamura JM. Biologic resurfacing of the glenoid using a meniscal allograft. *Tech Hand Up Extrem Surg.* 2006;10:145-149.
2. Krishnan SG, Reineck JR, Nowinski RJ, Harrison D, Burkhead WZ. Humeral hemiarthroplasty with biologic resurfacing of the glenoid for glenohumeral arthritis. Two to fifteen-year outcomes. *J Bone Joint Surg Am.* 2007;89:727-734.
3. Parsons IM, Millet PJ, Warner JP. Glenoid wear after shoulder hemiarthroplasty. *Clin Orthop Rel Res.* 2004; 421:120-125.
4. Creighton RA, Cole B, Nicholson G, Romeo A, Lorenz E. Effect of lateral meniscus allograft on shoulder articular contact areas and pressures. *J Shoulder Elbow Surg.* 2007;16:367-72.
5. Ball CM, Galatz LM, Yamaguchi K. Meniscal allograft interposition arthroplasty for the arthritic shoulder: description of a new surgical technique. *Tech Shoulder Elbow Surg.* 2001;2:247-254.
6. Weinstein DM, Bucchieri JS, Pollock RG, Flatow EL, Bigliani LU. Arthroscopic debridement of shoulder for osteoarthritis. *Arthroscopy.* 2000;16:471-476.

WHAT ARE YOUR INDICATIONS FOR REPAIR OF AN ACUTE PECTORALIS MAJOR TENDON TEAR AND WHAT IS YOUR PREFERRED METHOD OF FIXATION?

Christopher Dewing, MD
Matthew T. Provencher, MD, LCDR, MC, USNR

We have found that pectoralis major tendon tears occur most commonly during the bench press exercise, usually during the transition from an eccentric load to a concentric muscle contraction.[1] When evaluating a patient with a suspected pectoralis major tear, it is important to know the anatomy of the muscle-tendon unit and attachments in order to completely evaluate the muscle. The pectoralis major muscle has 2 main divisions; the superior portion is the clavicular head and takes its origin from the clavicle and superior aspect of the sternum, whereas the inferior division consists of the sternal head and has a broad origin from the inferior sternum, the external oblique, and the first 6 ribs. Wolfe[2] described the 2 divisions rotating 90 degrees as they coalesce to their tendinous insertion at the lateral aspect of the bicipital groove, leaving the fibers of the clavicular head inferior and anterior to those of the sternal head. Innervation is provided by the medial and lateral pectoral nerves: the medial nerve is to the lateral sternal head, the lateral nerve to the clavicular head and medial sternal head.[3]

When we are evaluating a suspected pectoralis major tear in the acute setting, usually defined as less than 6 weeks postinjury, patients present with pain, localized swelling/ecchymosis, and a webbed appearance to the axillary skin fold. Often the swelling is localized—either over the chest wall, signifying a muscle belly tear, or over the proximal arm, suggesting a musculotendinous tear at the insertion.[3] Patients will usually have diminished adduction and internal rotation strength compared with the noninjured side.

We always obtain a standard shoulder series to rule out bony avulsion fragments from the tendinous insertion. Usually we obtain a magnetic resonance imaging (MRI) of the chest wall to include the proximal humerus. This helps to characterize the tear as partial or complete and to define the location of the tear.[4]

Although classification systems for pectoralis major tears have been proposed,[5] we agree with defining the tear based on its location and extent.[3] Our indications for surgical repair are any complete tear and/or any partial tear resulting in significant weakness and deformity. Usually, patients with pectoralis major tears are young, physically active, and desire to return to a high level of activity. Studies have documented good to excellent results and near complete return of strength with surgical repair.[1] Nonsurgical treatment of complete tears has shown consistently poor results.[6]

 Our preferred surgical approach is to position the patient in the beach-chair position with the entire arm prepped free. We make a standard deltopectoral approach through an incision usually no more than 6 cm in length centered over the pectoralis major insertion area. We curve the distal aspect of the incision slightly lateral to allow for good visualization of the tendinous insertion. In many cases, the clavicular head will be intact and may be followed out to its humeral insertion, as a guide for the ruptured sternal head. Also, we have found that the anterior fascia over the sternal head may have to be incised before hematoma from the rupture will be encountered. In isolated tears of the sternal head, we look for the retracted tendon posterior to the clavicular fibers. It should be noted that the bicipital groove is just medial to the insertion of the pectoralis major on the humerus.

In the case of a tendinous avulsion, we carefully prepare the torn end of the tendon and use no. 5 nonabsorbable sutures in a whip-stitch fashion to secure the end of the tendon. We then use a 2-mm high-speed burr to prepare the insertion site. Initially we burr the cortical bone to a bleeding surface. We then use the burr to make a bone-trough[7] approximately 3 cm in vertical length and sufficiently deep to accommodate 3 to 5 equally spaced drill holes made by a 2-mm drill from anterior to lateral that will accommodate suture passage by a free needle. The grasping sutures can then be passed by Hewson ligature passer and tied down over the bone, ensuring excellent apposition of tendon to bone. The sutures are tightened with the arm in adduction and internal rotation.

If the tear is intramuscular and well proximal to the tendon insertion, we have had good success with placing nonabsorbable no. 5 modified Kessler grasping sutures in the proximal muscle.[8] These are placed in 3 layers—anterior fascia, middle muscle substance, and posterior fascia—to ensure excellent purchase of the full thickness of muscle belly. If adequate tendon is present, a free needle is used to suture the free ends to the tendon itself. If there is little or no healthy tendon stump left at the insertion, then we recommend proceeding with the trough and tunnel technique as described above.

For our postoperative rehabilitation, we use a sling and start Codman's exercises, and passive motion (flexion in adduction) for 4 weeks. We avoid external rotation beyond 30 degrees for 6 weeks.[8] We begin active range of motion (ROM) at 6 weeks to include abduction and external rotation, progressing to full active ROM at 10 to 12 weeks. Gentle strength training is allowed at 10 to 12 weeks. Push-ups and light bench press is allowed at the 6-month mark, with return to sport or heavy lifting labor when strength is approaching or equal to that of the noninjured extremity.

References

1. Bak K, Cameron EA, Henderson IJ. Rupture of the pectoralis major: a meta-analysis of 112 cases. *Knee Surg Sports Traumatol Arthrosc.* 2000;8:113-119.
2. Wolfe SW, Wickiewicz TL, Cavanaugh JT. Rupture of the pectoralis major muscle: an anatomic and clinical analysis. *Am J Sports Med.* 1992;20:587-593.
3. Petilon J, Carr DR, Sekiya JK, Unger DV. Pectoralis major muscle injuries: evaluation and management. *J Am Acad Orthop Surg.* 2005;13:59-68.
4. Connell DA, Potter HG, Sherman MF, et al. Injuries of the pectoralis major muscle: evaluation with MR imaging. *Radiology.* 1999;210:785-791.
5. Tietjen R. Closed injuries of the pectoralis major muscle. *J Trauma.* 1980;20:262-264.
6. Hanna CM, Glenny AB, Stanley SN, Caughey MA. Pectoralis major tears: comparison of surgical and conservative treatment. *Br J Sports Med.* 2001;35:202-206.
7. Kretzler HH Jr, Richardson AB. Rupture of the pectoralis major muscle. *Am J Sports Med.* 1989;17:453-458.
8. Schepsis AA, Grafe MW, Jones HP, Lemos MJ. Rupture of the pectoralis major muscle: outcome after repair of acute and chronic injuries. *Am J Sports Med.* 2000;28:9C-15C.

A 40-Year-Old Laborer Has Shoulder Pain. An Electromyograph Reveals Chronic Denervation of the Serratus Anterior Muscle Without Reinnervation. What Is Your Preferred Treatment for a Patient With Chronic Symptomatic Winging of the Shoulder Due to Serratus Anterior Palsy?

Christopher S. Ahmad, MD
John-Erik Bell, MD

When evaluating a patient with winging of the scapula, it is important to know that the most common cause is serratus anterior dysfunction secondary to long thoracic nerve injury, although other causes have been described. This can be painful and debilitating, and is often complicated by misdiagnosis and subsequent delay in appropriate treatment.[1] In fact, we feel that many patients with this condition undergo surgical procedures intended to treat an incorrect diagnosis.[2] Serratus anterior palsy has multiple etiologies, including acute penetrating or blunt trauma, iatrogenic injury from axillary dissection and mastectomy, Parsonage-Turner syndrome, or viral illness. It is important to identify the cause of the lesion because this will affect prognosis and timing of potential surgical intervention.

Figure 21-1. A 23-year-old female with over 2 years of post-traumatic refractory inferomedial periscapular pain and prominent scapular winging.

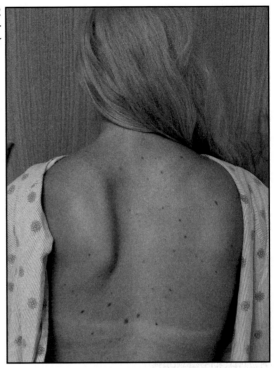

Patients with serratus anterior palsy typically present with periscapular pain, weakness, and pain with forward elevation, which is especially severe with prolonged activity. The pain is typically localized to muscles that antagonize the function of the serratus anterior, such as the rhomboids and levator scapulae, and can also be present in the scapulothoracic bursa. There are no other periscapular muscles that can effectively compensate for the function of the serratus anterior. The serratus anterior protracts and superiorly rotates the scapula and is responsible for keeping the scapula closely apposed to the chest wall during arm elevation. When weak, the inferior angle of the scapula rotates medially and superiorly, becoming prominent as it rotates away from the chest wall (Figure 21-1). The wall push-up test is ideal to test for serratus anterior weakness because it exacerbates this prominence. Resisted forward elevation will also typically accentuate winging. A cervical spine examination and thorough shoulder examination are also mandatory. Radiographs or more advanced imaging studies are typically not necessary, unless an unusual process is suspected, such as scapular osteochondroma or other neoplasm, or cervical spine etiology. The most important diagnostic tests are the electromyogram and nerve conduction studies, which are critical for both definitive diagnosis and subsequent management.

Fortunately, the majority of cases of acute serratus anterior palsy resolve spontaneously, but up to 25% become chronic, refractory to conservative treatments.[1,3,4] Nonoperative treatment consists of physical therapy focusing on maintaining range of motion, strengthening of the functional periscapular muscles, and occasionally the use of scapular stabilizing orthotics.[5] Spontaneous resolution typically occurs between 6 and 9 months for traumatic cases and within 2 years for atraumatic cases.[1] When these intervals have passed and the dysfunction and pain persist, surgical treatment can be very successful.

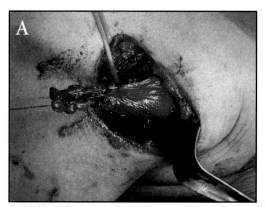

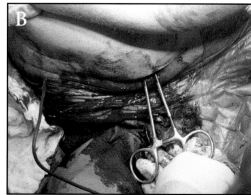

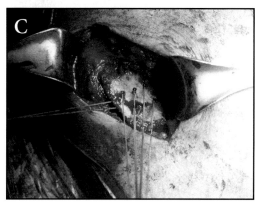

Figure 21-2. (A) Sternal head of pectoralis major is released from its humeral insertion and a nonabsorbable no. 2 suture is placed in Krackow configuration to secure it. (B) Pectoralis is transferred along the chest wall posteriorly to the inferior angle of the scapula using a long curved clamp. (C) The transferred pectoralis tendon is secured to the inferior angle of the scapula through drill holes.

We prefer a dynamic stabilization surgery such as the split pectoralis major tendon transfer. This procedure is well described in the literature and has shown excellent results in published studies.[3,6-9] In this procedure, the patient is positioned in the lateral decubitus position, supported on a beanbag. A concealed axillary incision is used, spanning 4 cm in the axillary skin fold directed toward the lateral border of the coracoid process. The deltopectoral interval is identified and the cephalic vein is mobilized laterally with the deltoid. The sternal head of the pectoralis major, which lies deep to the clavicular head, is isolated, detached from its humeral insertion, and mobilized medially. It is secured with a no. 2 nonabsorbable suture passed with a Krackow configuration (Figure 21-2). It is important to avoid damage to the long head of the biceps during release from the humerus and it is critical to mobilize no further than 8 cm medially to avoid damage to the lateral pectoral nerve, which has been reported to result in recurrent winging after transfer.[10,11] Appropriate release and mobilization will typically yield sufficient tendon length to reach the medial border of the inferior scapula primarily without the need for spanning soft-tissue graft. A second 4-cm longitudinal incision is then made posteriorly at the inferomedial border of the scapula. This is carried to fascia, and the soft-tissues posteriorly (infraspinatus and teres minor), medially (rhomboid major), and anteriorly (serratus anterior and subscapularis) are subperiosteally elevated off the scapula, skeletonizing the inferomedial angle. The tunnel for tendon passage is created bluntly, staying immediately against the chest wall to avoid damage to the more lateral nerves and vessels in the axilla. A curved Kelly is passed from posterior to anterior to retrieve the sutures in the pectoralis tendon and bring them into the posterior incision. The tendon is then secured to the scapula through bone tunnels with suture fixation.

Alternative treatments for serratus anterior palsy include static stabilization procedures, which involve using tendon graft to secure the scapula to the vertebral column or to an adjacent rib, the so-called "loose" scapulopexy. We do not prefer these types of procedures because they do not restore normal scapulothoracic mechanics in the way the dynamic pectoralis major transfer does and can potentially restrict scapulothoracic, and in turn, overall shoulder motion significantly. Although scapulothoracic fusion is another alternative, we generally reserve this as a salvage procedure only for failed dynamic transfers or conditions in which dynamic transfer is not possible due to global shoulder girdle dysfunction (ie, fascioscapulohumeral dystrophy or diffuse brachial plexus injury).

References

1. Wiater JM, Flatow EL. Long thoracic nerve injury. *Clin Orthop.* 1999;368:17-27.
2. Warner JJ, Navarro RA. Serratus anterior dysfunction. Recognition and treatment. *Clin Orthop.* 1998;349:139-148.
3. Connor PM, Yamaguchi K, Manifold SG, Pollock RG, Flatow EL, Bigliani LU. Split pectoralis major transfer for serratus anterior palsy. *Clin Orthop Relat Res.* 1997;341:134-142.
4. Post M. Pectoralis major transfer for winging of the scapula. *J Shoulder Elbow Surg.* 1995;4(1 Pt 1):1-9.
5. Watson CJ, Schenkman M. Physical therapy management of isolated serratus anterior muscle paralysis. *Phys Ther.* 1995;75:194-202.
6. Noerdlinger MA, Cole BJ, Stewart M, Post M. Results of pectoralis major transfer with fascia lata autograft augmentation for scapula winging. *J Shoulder Elbow Surg.* 2002;11:345-350.
7. Perlmutter GS, Leffert RD. Results of transfer of the pectoralis major tendon to treat paralysis of the serratus anterior muscle. *J Bone Joint Surg Am.* 1999;81:377-384.
8. Povacz P, Resch H. Dynamic stabilization of winging scapula by direct split pectoralis major transfer: a technical note. *J Shoulder Elbow Surg.* 2000;9:76-78.
9. Steinmann SP, Wood MB. Pectoralis major transfer for serratus anterior paralysis. *J Shoulder Elbow Surg.* 2003;12:555-560.
10. Klepps SJ, Goldfarb C, Flatow E, Galatz LM, Yamaguchi K. Anatomic evaluation of the subcoracoid pectoralis major transfer in human cadavers. *J Shoulder Elbow Surg.* 2001;10:453-459.
11. Litts CS, Hennigan SP, Williams GR. Medial and lateral pectoral nerve injury resulting in recurrent scapular winging after pectoralis major transfer: a case report. *J Shoulder Elbow Surg.* 2000;9:347-349.

How Do You Manage A Symptomatic Superior Labrum Anterior to Posterior II Tear In Someone Older Than 45 Years of Age? Tenotomy, Repair, or Tenodesis?

Clifford G. Rios, MD
Robert A. Arciero, MD
Anthony A. Romeo, MD
Augustus D. Mazzocca, MD

Before considering management of a symptomatic superior labrum anterior to posterior (SLAP) II tear, you need to first identify and confirm this as the source of the patient's symptoms. A SLAP lesion most commonly is associated with other intra-articular pathology, such as partial or complete rotator cuff tears, impingement, and Bankart lesions in younger patients.[1] In our experience, it is rare that a patient over 40 years old will have a SLAP lesion as the primary cause of his symptoms. Failing to diagnose and address the primary pathology while repairing an asymptomatic SLAP lesion will fail to relieve the patient's symptoms and puts him at risk for significant loss of motion. Thus, it is critical that you perform a thorough history and complete shoulder examination to rule out other causes of your patient's symptoms; the SLAP lesion is almost a diagnosis of exclusion.

We suspect SLAP lesions in a younger patient who presents with pain and mechanical symptoms such as grinding or clicking, particularly with overhead activities. A history of a traction or compression injury also suggests a SLAP lesion. On examination, shoulder pain localized to the lateral arm associated with weakness with scaption or belly press suggests the rotator cuff is the pain generator. Pain with biceps provocative tests (eg, Speed's, O'Brien's, SLAP compression) suggests a biceps or SLAP etiology. These issues must be identified and treated appropriately. We find a glenohumeral joint injection of

Figure 22-1. This arthroscopic image demonstrates detachment and fraying of the anterior glenoid labrum extending posteriorly and including the biceps anchor. There is also hyperemia of the proximal biceps tendon.

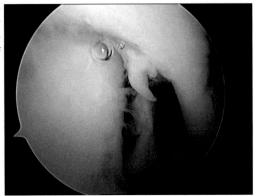

10 cc lidocaine, with or without steroid, helpful in confirming an intra-articular source of the patient's symptoms. This injection will alleviate symptoms attributable to the proximal biceps due to continuity between its tendon sheath and the glenohumeral joint. The patient is kept in the room for an extra few minutes while we reexamine the shoulder to make sure there is no pain. A magnetic resonance arthrogram (MRI arthogram) also helps us further delineate between other potential causes of the patient's symptoms. Still, diagnosing a SLAP tear can be an arduous task, and even after a thorough history and physical examination, diagnostic arthroscopy remains the only way to make a definitive diagnosis.

Type II SLAP lesions are characterized by detachment of the superior labrum and biceps anchor from the superior glenoid[2] (Figure 22-1). In the face of an unstable labral tear, debridement alone is associated with suboptimal outcomes.[3] We treat these patients individually and attempt to tailor the operative management of SLAP lesions to the patient's vocational or recreational demands, and consider hand dominance and medical comorbidities as well. If the patient is a physiologically young laborer who needs to return to work as soon as possible, we perform a subpectoral biceps tenodesis and leave the SLAP lesion alone. Alternatively, we have also fixed a SLAP and performed a biceps tenodesis, and rehabilitate the patient as if only the tenodesis was done. In the nonlaborer, nonoverhead athlete who can avoid strenuous activity for several months, we would fix the SLAP tear and perform a biceps tenodesis. If the patient were an overhead athlete, we would fix the SLAP and not perform a biceps tenodesis. These patients are at risk for biceps tendonitis, which typically responds well to an intra-articular corticosteroid injection. We reserve biceps tenotomy for elderly patients, or sedentary patients with diabetes or obesity. We have not had patients present with symptoms of glenohumeral instability following biceps tenodesis or tenotomy.

We perform this procedure with the patient in the beach-chair position. We use 3 portals—a standard posterior portal and two anterior portals. We place an anterosuperior cannula just anterior to the biceps tendon, and an anteroinferior cannula just above the superior border of the subscapularis tendon. All canulae are 8.25 mm to allow easier passage of curved instruments. Finally, we will use the Port of Wilmington placed 1 cm inferior and 1 cm anterior from the posterolateral corner of the acromion to help place anchors. The technique we use reattaches the type II lesion to the glenoid with a push-in–type suture anchor. We place 1 anchor anterior and 1 or 2 anchors posterior to the biceps origin

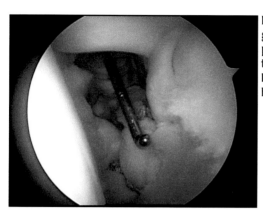

Figure 22-2. This SLAP lesion was secured to the glenoid with 1 anchor anterior and 2 anchors posterior to the biceps origin. Before placing these anchors, it is critical that you create a bleeding bony bed to which the labrum may heal.

(Figure 22-2). Before placing these anchors, it is critical that you create a bleeding bony bed to which the labrum may heal. We typically use a SLAP burr, meniscal rasp, or shaver to accomplish this. If we perform a biceps tenodesis, we prefer a subpectoral tenodesis to the arthroscopic method for several reasons.[4] First, the anatomy is clearly defined and the length-tension relationship of the biceps can be reproduced easily. Second, this technique removes the biceps from the intertuberular groove, which is lined by synovium and can be a continued source of inflammation and pain. Lastly, it provides excellent stability with interference and suture-anchor construction.

We like to move these patients early in the postoperative period. Communication with your physical therapist is critical and preserving your patient's range of motion (ROM) following a SLAP repair is of utmost importance. Stiffness is a considerable problem and the patient will be disappointed with a stiff shoulder, regardless of the quality of your repair/tenodesis. Our typical approach to the patient who has had a SLAP repair is to have patients wear a sling for comfort for 2 to 4 weeks and discontinue it as their pain level subsides. We encourage gentle passive and active-assisted ROM during the immediate days postoperatively. External and internal rotation begins around week 3 and full ROM is allowed by week 8. Elbow ROM and grip strengthening can progress as tolerated without concern for the biceps tenodesis. We allow patients to return to full activity at around 12 weeks. This represents a conservative rehabilitation protocol. If we performed a biceps tenodesis and did not repair the SLAP tear, we allow earlier motion if needed such that many tenodesis patients can resume activity as tolerated at week 2, but they are informed of the risks. In our practice, postoperative activity is typically dictated by the procedures that have been performed in conjunction with the biceps tenodesis or tenotomy.

References

1. Snyder SJ, Banas MP, Karzel RP. An analysis of 140 injuries to the superior glenoid labrum. *J Shoulder Elbow Surg.* 1995;4:243-248.
2. Snyder SJ, Karzel RP, Del Pizzo, Ferkel RD, Friedman MJ. SLAP lesions of the shoulder. *Arthroscopy.* 1990;6: 274-279.
3. Cordasco FA, Steinmann S, Flatow EL, Bigliani LU. Arthroscopic treatment of glenoid labral tears. *Am J Sports Med.* 1993;21:425-431.
4. Mazzocca AD, Rios CG, Romeo AA, Arciero RA. Subpectoral biceps tenodesis with interference screw fixation. *Arthroscopy.* 2005;21:896.

What Are the Indications for Conservative Treatment Versus Core Decompression Versus Arthroplasty in Avascular Necrosis of the Humeral Head?

Sumant G. "Butch" Krishnan, MD
Kenneth C. Lin, MD

After the femoral head, the humeral head is the second most common site of osteonecrosis or avascular necrosis (AVN) (Figure 23-1). Unfortunately, once the blood supply to an involved area of the humeral head is compromised and bone death occurs, there is no reversal. Progressive AVN leads to eventual subchondral collapse and glenohumeral arthritis. Hence the appropriate management of humeral head AVN involves early suspicion and diagnosis in an attempt to preserve the shoulder joint.[1]

AVN is classically "staged" by the Cruess modification of the Arlet-Ficat classification system (Table 23-1). Clinical and radiographic evaluation of humeral head AVN allows for an individualized approach to management.[1] We closely evaluate range of motion (ROM) in comparison to the opposite (usually uninvolved) shoulder. In each patient with suspected AVN, our standard plain radiographic views (anteroposterior views in neutral and external rotation, axillary-lateral view, and supraspinatus outlet view) are combined with magnetic resonance imaging (MRI) in order to evaluate the extent of the necrosis. In addition to nonoperative measures such as nonsteroidal anti-inflammatory drugs (NSAIDs) and physical therapy, operative treatment for AVN involves either reduction in intraosseous pressure (core decompression), replacement of the diseased head (hemiarthroplasty), or replacement of the entire joint (total shoulder arthroplasty).

Figure 23-1. Anteroposterior radiograph demonstrating AVN of the humeral head with subchondral collapse.

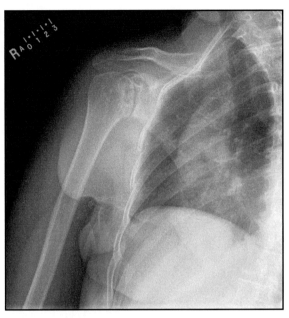

Table 23-1

Staging System for Avascular Necrosis of the Humeral Head

STAGE 1 AVN: Normal radiographs.
STAGE 2 AVN: Architecture of humeral head preserved with sclerotic changes visible.
STAGE 3 AVN: Subchondral collapse of humeral head with loss of sphericity.
STAGE 4 AVN: Progressive collapse of the humeral head with degenerative arthrosis and joint space narrowing.
STAGE 5 AVN: Degenerative arthrosis in both humeral head and glenoid with loss of joint space.

For early stage disease prior to subchondral collapse (stages 0, 1, and 2), joint preservation techniques remain paramount. Although a short trial (6-week increments) of simple nonoperative exercises and activity modification may be initiated, we consider these early stages as the shoulder "at risk," and hence utilize aggressive nonoperative treatment in conjunction with arthroscopic modifications of the core decompression procedure as soon as possible.[2] Peer-reviewed literature has demonstrated successful clinical and radiographic evidence supporting the use of core decompression in retarding the progression of AVN in these early precollapse stages. We combine clinical history with MRI to confirm this diagnosis and proceed with management. Patients are counseled that although core decompression indeed reduces pain, the long-term results beyond 5 to 10 years remain unknown (Figure 23-2). We perform this procedure in the upright beach-chair position, under both arthroscopic and fluoroscopic control. A standard anterior cruciate ligament tibial targeting guide is utilized through a standard anterior glenohumeral arthroscopic portal in order to confirm appropriate placement under the softened and sometimes fibrillated area of cartilage (most commonly in the anterosuperolateral humeral head). Under fluoroscopic imaging, a guide pin is placed through a

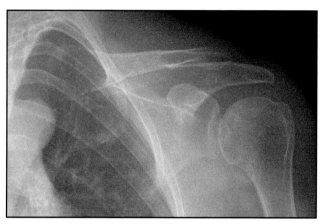

Figure 23-2. Anteroposterior radiograph 5 years after arthroscopic assisted core decompression. Humeral head architecture is still preserved.

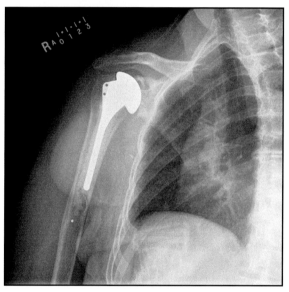

Figure 23-3. Hemiarthroplasty for AVN.

small incision on the lateral arm and advanced to the subchondral surface—confirming lack of articular penetration via the arthroscope in the joint. This pin is over-reamed with a standard 6- or 7-mm acorn reamer depending on patient size, taking care not to advance the pin into the joint. Aggressive postoperative management includes no immobilization, immediate terminal ROM and stretching exercises, scapular stabilization strengthening, and emphasis on glenohumeral and scapulothoracic flexibilities.

When the subchondral plate has collapsed (stage 3 and beyond), we do not recognize the benefit of joint preservation surgery. These patients are managed with a more prolonged course of conservative management (3-month increments) with heavy emphasis on glenohumeral flexibility and activity modification. Some patients will respond to these measures and may be satisfied with their shoulders, although disease progression remains inevitable. For these "early responders," we recommend follow-up at 3- to 6-month intervals in order to continue measures to alleviate symptoms (judicious use of corticosteroid injections, alterations in the NSAID regimen, etc).

If all nonoperative attempts are exhausted due to persistent disabling symptoms, we proceed to arthroplasty as our operative management (Figure 23-3). The decision for hemiarthroplasty versus total shoulder arthroplasty must be carefully considered based on 3 parameters: (1) stage of the disease and the joint collapse, (2) status of the soft-tissue contractures associated with this disease, and (3) age of the patient.[3]

References

1. Wolfe CJ, Taylor-Butler KL. Avascular necrosis. *Arch Fam Med.* 2000;9:291-294.
2. Chapman C, Mattern C, Levine WN. Arthroscopically assisted core decompression of the proximal humerus for avascular necrosis. *Arthroscopy.* 2004;20:1003-1006.
3. Mansat P, Huser L, Mansat M, et al. Shoulder arthroplasty for atraumatic avascular necrosis of the humeral head: nineteen shoulders followed up for a mean of seven years. *J Shoulder Elbow Surg.* 2005;14:114-120.

A 70-Year-Old Patient Is Referred With a Magnetic Resonance Imaging Report That States a Supraspinatus Tear and Significant Degenerative Changes of the Glenohumeral Joint. Do You Counsel the Patient for Rotator Cuff Repair, Total Shoulder Replacement With Cuff Repair, or a Reverse Shoulder Replacement?

Michael L. Pearl, MD

When I evaluate a patient with both a rotator cuff tear and degenerative changes of the glenohumeral joint, I want to make sure that I have all of my preoperative information. Radiology reports of degenerative changes have ranged for me from almost insignificant to total loss of joint space. Similarly, magnetic resonance imaging (MRI) reports of rotator cuff tears don't give the full picture of the rotator cuff status. I recommend reviewing the actual radiographic and MRI images to determine the level of osteoarthritis, determine the size of the tear, as well as atrophy of the rotator cuff muscles. I need to examine the patient and see the actual film to define what condition I am dealing with. For the sake of discussion, let's suppose that it is osteoarthritis with the associated finding of a supraspinatus tear.

Based on the available literature, if a supraspinatus tear is present with significant osteoarthritis, I would only recommend a repair attempt in the setting of rotator cuff tendon

Figure 24-1. Preoperative MRI.

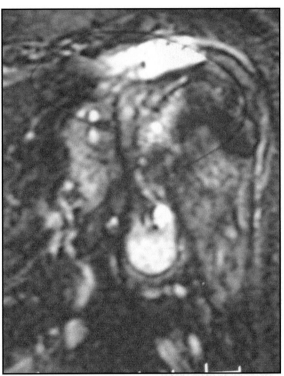

ruptures that result in instability of the glenohumeral joint. By this I mean superior migration of the humeral head in relationship to the center of the glenoid. The Mayo approach now is to treat only those tendon ruptures that result in instability. This is consistent with the most relevant experience in the literature from a French multicenter study published in 2002 in which patients that had an isolated supraspinatus tear at surgery did equally well with or without repair.[1] Since the presentation and publication of this work, that has been my practice as well and I have not seen any reason to alter this practice.

However, if the symptoms are also attributable to significant glenohumeral osteoarthritis, I would plan for a total shoulder arthroplasty (TSA). If physical examination of the patient demonstrates moderate or greater external rotation power, and an isolated supraspinatus tear is discovered either on preoperative MRI (I rarely get MRIs preoperatively for osteoarthritis) or at surgery, I will not repair it and proceed with an unconstrained shoulder arthroplasty. So, if a patient planned for TSA has a well-centered head in the frontal plane (on anteroposterior [AP] projection), I would proceed with a TSA. Doing otherwise also complicates the rehabilitation considerably because I encourage early active motion.

One case that comes to mind is a 74-year-old woman sent to me for "cuff-tear arthropathy." Her primary care doctor had obtained an MRI early on and referred her to an orthopedic specialist after seeing the radiologist's finding of rotator cuff tear (Figures 24-1 and 24-2). The orthopedist referring her to me was clear that it was an arthritic problem but figured that these 2 findings meant that she had cuff-tear arthropathy. Despite her apprehension, she had a successful TSA (Figure 24-3) and a couple of years later returned for the same operation on her other shoulder.

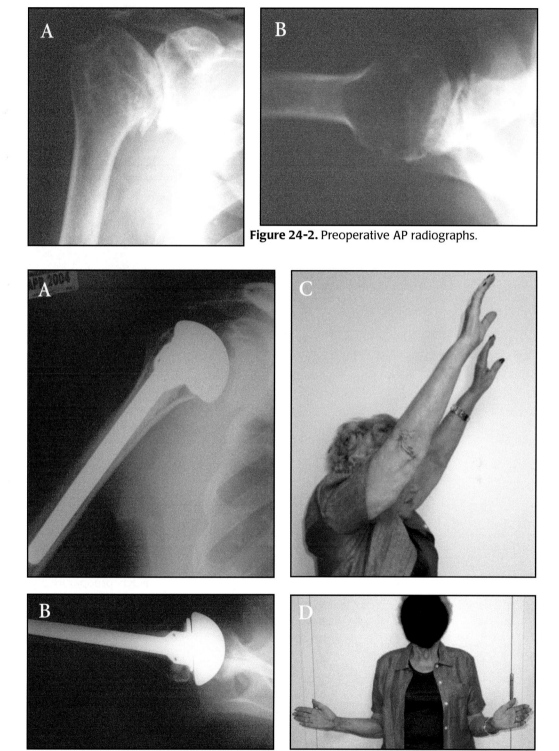

Figure 24-2. Preoperative AP radiographs.

Figure 24-3. One-year postoperative radiographs and motion.

An isolated supraspinatus tear in the setting of glenohumeral osteoarthritis is not a contraindication to a TSA. If the tendon is severely involved on imaging studies and their physical examination findings corroborate a profound weakness in external rotation (and usually other motions as well), then I would counsel the patient for a reverse TSA, given the significant rotator cuff dysfunction.

Reference

1. Edwards TB, Boulahia A, Kempf JF, et al. The influence of rotator cuff disease on the results of shoulder arthro-plasty for primary osteoarthritis: results of a multicenter study. *J Bone Joint Surg Am.* 2002;84A:2240-2248.

25

HOW DO YOU WORK UP THE CLINICAL SITUATION OF ASEPTIC LOOSENING VERSUS POSSIBLE OCCULT INFECTION IN A TOTAL SHOULDER WITH INCOMPLETE 2-MM LUCENT LINES AROUND THE CEMENTED GLENOID?

Gregory P. Nicholson, MD

Almost all cemented total shoulder arthroplasties (TSAs) utilizing polyethylene glenoid components will develop lucent lines or incomplete lucent lines around the glenoid component over time.[1] This obviously does not mean that it is necessarily symptomatic or infected. When working up this situation of lucent lines around the glenoid component, one of the big factors to take into account is the time course involved. How far out from surgery has the lucent line appeared? If the lucent lines have appeared within 1 year of the TSA, this is more concerning for infection than aseptic loosening.

Most patients are asymptomatic. Thus, a good history is important. Has the patient noted a gradual onset of pain in the shoulder where before he was were pain-free? Has he been doing heavy labor or suffered a trauma or a fall that might have contributed to the lucent line appearance? Has he had recent surgery in other musculoskeletal areas or abdominal surgery that might have led to hematogenous seating of this arthroplasty?

Physical examination is important, especially in a serial examination fashion. Gradual increasing pain and loss of function is obviously another concerning factor for infection when there are incomplete lucent lines.

Good radiographs are important. A true anteroposterior (AP) of the glenohumeral joint to try to image the cemented glenoid component face-on is important (Figure 25-1).

Figure 25-1. True AP of the glenohumeral joint, imaging the glenoid component at 90 degrees. Note the lucency around the inferior peg.

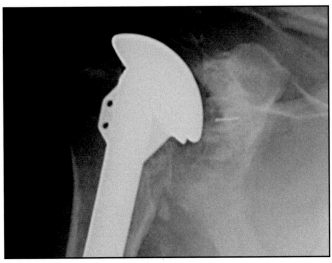

This is the best way to determine the cement mantle and the bone-cement interface. This is important for both pegged designs and keel design. An axillary x-ray is important to determine if there has been bone resorption under the posterior aspect of the glenoid or if there is poor bone support underneath this area that might lead to mechanical aseptic loosening. It can evaluate for excessive retroversion of the implant as well.

Laboratory work-up is important. I would recommend a C-reactive protein, a sedimentation rate, and a complete blood count. If the C-reactive protein and sedimentation rate are both elevated, it is concerning for a possible occult infection.[2] It must be kept in mind, however, that an occult infection can be present with normal laboratory values, but it is certainly less likely.

The advanced imaging study that I prefer is an arthrogram–computed tomography (CT) scan. Many times fluid is not obtainable within the joint in this clinical situation but a possible aspiration could be attempted. If that fluid is obtained, then it can be sent for cell count, culture, and sensitivity. However, the value of the arthrogram-CT scan is to place dye within the glenohumeral joint. This will determine if there is a rotator cuff tear that is creating abnormal biomechanical forces across the glenoid component. It will also give the surgeon a qualitative assessment of the muscle bellies of the rotator cuff and the status of the subscapularis. Most importantly, if there is dye that goes behind the glenoid component, behind the cement mantle around the pegs or the keel, this would point toward a loose glenoid component (Figure 25-2). Many times, there can be an incomplete 2-mm lucent line, but that is fibrous tissue and a stable interface and the dye cannot leak behind the component. In an infected situation, most likely the dye is going to completely surround the component and outline the bone-cement interface early. The CT scan will also give better determination of the bone support behind the glenoid component itself.

With that information, a recommendation can be made to the patient. Typically, if an incomplete <2-mm line is found and the patient has no pain and he is functioning well, serial examinations and observations would be recommended and a new x-ray would be taken in 4 months to compare to the previous x-ray to document progression of the lucent line.

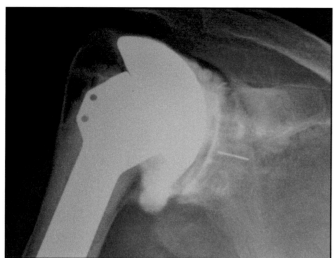

Figure 25-2. The same patient as in Figure 25-1, with an arthrogram-CT scan. Note the dye behind the glenoid component and around the pegs. This was an aseptically loose glenoid component.

Summary

An incomplete 2-mm line around a cemented glenoid component within the first year of a TSA is worrisome for infection. The work-up should consist of a good history and physical examination, and good plain radiographs in the true AP plane of the glenohumeral joint and the axillary plane. C-reactive protein and sedimentation rate should be obtained and potentially an arthrogram-CT scan performed. If the C-reactive protein and sedimentation rate are elevated, it is more worrisome for occult infection.

If the lucent lines have developed over a longer period of time, for example in the third or fifth year after a TSA and the patient is completely asymptomatic, this is a situation that is followed clinically. Serial x-rays at every 6 months to 1 year should be obtained along with good documentation of the patient's pain level, functional level, and range of motion. Clear communication between the surgeon and the patient about the meaning or significance of incomplete 2-mm lucent lines around a cemented glenoid component should be undertaken to avoid misinterpretation and misunderstanding by the patient.

References

1. Pfahler M, Jena F, Neyton F, Sirveaux F, Mole D. Hemiarthroplasty versus total shoulder prosthesis: Results of cemented glenoid components. *J Shoulder Elbow Surg.* 2006;15:154-163.
2. Greidanus NV, Masri BA, Garbuz DS, et al. Use of erythrocyte sedimentation rate and C-reactive protein level to diagnose infection before revision total knee arthroplasty. *J Bone Joint Surg.* 2007;89A:1409-1416.

A PATIENT WITH SHOULDER DEGENERATIVE JOINT DISEASE AND IN NEED OF A SHOULDER ARTHROPLASTY HAS A SIGNIFICANT LOSS OF EXTERNAL ROTATION AT THE SIDE OF −15 DEGREES UNDER ANESTHESIA. WHAT ARE THE OPTIONS FOR SUBSCAPULARIS MANAGEMENT, AND WHAT APPROACH WOULD BE APPROPRIATE?

Michael L. Pearl, MD

This is an area that generates much debate. Subscapularis management is a hot topic, with several authors now recommending techniques of lesser tuberosity osteotomy as a way of obtaining more secure fixation, restoration of the anatomy, and hopefully optimal subscapularis function.[1,2] The debate centers on 2 issues: (1) do you need to do this in order to achieve subscapularis function, and (2) can you do this in the face of an internal rotation contracture?

First, a quick review of the techniques out there. Dr. Neer's original method was a Z-plasty lengthening of subscapularis to obtain greater external rotation range. Observations that the tissue left behind was often insubstantial, especially in the rheumatoid patient, led to interest in simply detaching the subscapularis from the bone as far lateral as possible, then resuturing it more medially at the osteotomy site. Two things intervened, challenging the need for either of these techniques: (1) we have improved methods for restoring the articular anatomy now (better implants) so we less often need to have a longer subscapularis; and (2) clinical studies are showing that subscapularis dysfunction is not uncommon after total shoulder arthoplasty (TSA). Hence the emergence of the other 2 alternatives—a lesser tuberosity osteotomy or simply doing a tenotomy and resuturing the tendon anatomically.

I have used all techniques. Like most who have done a lesser tuberosity osteotomy, I have been impressed with the solidity of fixation. However, I was not impressed by a marked improvement in my patient's ability to internally rotate. The ability to "lift off," if you will, seems much more related to the passive range of motion in internal rotation in my patients, so I have abandoned the lesser tuberosity osteotomy. In addition, as I press-fit most of my humeral stems, I am concerned about any technique that might compromise the proximal ring of bone and how it may impact on the initial fixation of the implant.

So what to do in the face of a profound internal rotation contracture, which for me is 0 degrees or less? I once thought that an anatomic reconstruction of the articular anatomy would take care of the problem, but I no longer believe that. Patients with long-standing contractures have shortened muscles, and sometimes restoration of the articular surfaces increases the size of the joint. In order to leave the operative room with at least 40 degrees of external rotation in all patients, we must be prepared to do something when the situation calls for it.

Dr. Matsen showed almost 2 decades ago that you get about 30 degrees of external rotation for every centimeter of subscapularis lengthening. I no longer do Z-plasty lengthenings and I prefer not to reattach the subscapularis to the medial osteotomy site, as I think it interferes with passive range of motion. Now, in every case, I do a very lateral tenotomy of the subscapularis tendon with the intention to repair it anatomically at the end of the case. This involved tendon-to-tendon sutures and sutures through bone tunnels if there is an insufficient tendon stump remaining. If the shoulder does not have a comfortable 30 to 40 degrees of passive external rotation with the arm at the side with this type of repair, I will suture the tendon more medially.

References

1. Gerber C, Yian EH, Pfirrmann CAW, Zumstein MA, Werner CML. Subscapularis muscle function and structure after total shoulder replacement with lesser tuberosity osteotomy and repair. *J Bone Joint Surg Am.* 2005;87:1739-1745.
2. Ponce BA, Ahluwalia RS, Mazzocca AD, et al. Biomechanical and clinical evaluation of a novel lesser tuberosity repair technique in total shoulder arthroplasty. *J Bone Joint Surg Am.* 2005;87(Suppl 2):1-8.

WHAT ARE THE RELATIVE INDICATIONS FOR REVERSE TOTAL SHOULDER ARTHROPLASTY?

Michael L. Pearl, MD

The absolute indication for reverse total shoulder arthoplasty (TSA) is rotator cuff rupture with glenohumeral arthrosis and pseudoparalysis of the arm.[1] In other words, patients who cannot raise their arms greater than 80 degrees or so, usually accompanied by pain and anterosuperior escape of the humeral head. There are other patients with conditions that may benefit from a reverse TSA, but these must be considered relative indications. For example, patients with cuff tear arthropathy that have weak elevation associated with pain may be best served by a reverse TSA instead of a hemiarthroplasty if they are otherwise age appropriate (>70 years old), so long as the risks have been discussed.

Other situations for which there are no other surgical answers compel consideration of the reverse TSA as well. Post fracture sequelae, with or without prior open reduction and internal fixation (ORIF) or hemiarthroplasty, that have arthrosis and diminished cuff function from tuberosity involvement in the fracture present many patients for whom reverse TSA is a consideration. Often, these patients are younger than 70 years old. Surgery is riskier in the postoperative setting, especially after failed hemiarthroplasty, but many of these patients can be returned to a higher level of function after conversion to a reverse TSA.

Patients with compromised glenoid bone stock and marked rotator cuff dysfunction may be relatively indicated for a reverse TSA. It is unclear how much glenoid bone is necessary at this point to implant a reverse successfully, but much of the fixation comes from the scapular body. On the other end of the spectrum, patients with fairly healthy glenohumeral cartilage may have nearly complete loss of rotator cuff function and be unable to raise their arms (pseudoparalysis). If soft-tissue procedures are unable to restore shoulder function, no other option exists for these patients other than the reverse.

Reference

1. Sirveaux F, Favard L, Oudet D, et al. Grammont inverted total shoulder arthroplasty in the treatment of gleno-humeral osteoarthritis with massive rupture of the cuff. Results of a multicentre study of 80 shoulders. *J Bone Joint Surg Br.* 2004;86:388-395.

QUESTION 28

THERE IS ATROPHY OF THE TRAPEZIUS AFTER LYMPH NODE BIOPSY 18 MONTHS AGO IN THE POSTERIOR CERVICAL TRIANGLE. WHAT ARE THE SURGICAL OPTIONS AND TECHNIQUES TO ADDRESS TRAPEZIUS MUSCLE PALSY?

Scot A. Youngblood, MD

Although trapezius muscle palsy is rare, the most common cause is injury to the spinal accessory nerve during a surgical procedure. Such iatrogenic injury has occurred after lymph node dissection, cervical mass excisional biopsy, radical neck dissection, external jugular vein catheterization, and carotid endarterectomy. Blunt and penetrating trauma are relatively rare causes of trapezius palsy. The spinal accessory nerve (cranial nerve XI) lies on the floor of the posterior cervical triangle and is vulnerable to injury. It is a pure motor nerve, and provides the sole innervation to the trapezius muscle. Trapezius palsy presents clinically with shoulder girdle drooping, neckline asymmetry, lateral scapular displacement and winging, and weakness and pain with forward elevation and abduction. One of the greatest challenges in treatment is actually recognizing the disorder—one study noted 14 of 22 patients referred were originally misdiagnosed.[1]

Initial nonoperative treatment consists of nonsteroidal anti-inflammatory medications, transcutaneous nerve stimulation, and physical therapy for range of motion (ROM) and strengthening. One goal of therapy is to prevent the development of adhesive capsulitis, a condition commonly found in these patients. If the patient is low-demand or sedentary, such nonoperative therapy may be sufficient. Such therapy is usually unsuccessful in the active patient, as the remaining scapular muscles possess inadequate bulk and mechanical advantage to properly compensate for trapezius function.

Patients who have demonstrated no clinical improvement within 3 months after injury are candidates for operative intervention. One recent study recommended surgical exploration with neurolysis, direct repair, or nerve grafting as appropriate for lesions present less than 12 months.[2] Lesions present greater than 12 but less than 20 months should be explored and undergo intraoperative stimulation, with nerve surgery or reconstructive muscle transfer performed as appropriate. Spontaneous lesions, those after a radical neck dissection, or those present greater than 20 months should be considered for a reconstructive procedure.

Multiple reconstructive procedures to compensate for trapezius function have been proposed. The Dewar-Harris procedure stabilized the medial portion of the scapula to the spinous processes of the thoracic spine with fascia lata graft, combined with the lateral transfer of the insertion of the levator scapulae.[3] Unfortunately, this and other such reconstructions have been associated with unsatisfactory stretching and failure with time.

In contrast to these static fascial reconstructions, the more dynamic triple muscle transfer described by Eden and Lange is associated with better outcomes, and is the most commonly used reconstruction.[1,2] It effectively substitutes for the 3 functional parts of the trapezius, by transferring 3 muscles laterally on the scapula. The levator scapulae is transferred to the lateral spine of the scapula, replacing the upper portion of the trapezius that upwardly rotates and elevates the scapula. The rhomboid minor and a portion of the rhomboid major replace the middle portion of the trapezius that stabilizes and adducts the scapula. The rhomboid major replaces the lower portion of the trapezius that downwardly rotates and depresses the scapula.

For the Eden-Lange procedure, the patient is placed in the lateral decubitus position, with the operative arm draped free for manipulation. A longitudinal incision parallel and just medial to the medial border of the scapula is created. The atrophied trapezius is transected medially close to its origin from the spinous processes, thus protecting the underlying rhomboids and levator scapulae. These 3 muscles are then dissected out from each other, as well as freeing them medially and proximally to facilitate their lateral transfer. The 3 muscle insertions on the medial scapula are then released with an osteotome, with a thin wafer of bone attached. The levator scapulae is then transferred to the lateral aspect of the scapular spine, approximately 5 to 7 cm from the posterolateral corner of the acromion. This is performed utilizing transosseous sutures through the scapular spine itself. The rhomboids are then transferred laterally onto the scapular body. Although the classic description involves attaching both to the scapula below the spine, a recent modification has been proposed involving attachment of the rhomboid minor to the supraspinatus fossa, whereas the rhomboid major is attached below the scapular spine, to the infraspinatus fossa.[1] The spinati muscles are then imbricated over the repaired muscles. After a period of immobilization, gentle active and passive ROM exercises are initiated.

Results of the Eden-Lange procedure are mixed in the literature. The largest series of 22 cases reported 13 excellent, 6 satisfactory, and 3 unsatisfactory overall results as scored by the American Shoulder and Elbow Surgeons Shoulder Evaluation Form.[1] Nineteen of these patients had no pain at rest and slight pain or discomfort after strenuous activity, whereas 3 had unsatisfactory relief of their pain. Another more recent series of seven patients reported 3 excellent, 1 good, and 3 poor results utilizing criteria such as ROM, pain, motor strength testing, and subjective patient satisfaction.[2] Factors predictive of a poor result were patient age greater than 50, a prior radical neck dissection, penetrating injury, or a spontaneous palsy.

In general, the results of nerve surgery are superior to a nonanatomical salvage reconstructive procedure. Operative intervention is recommended after 3 months of no clinical improvement and evidence of denervation potentials (fibrillations and sharp waves) on electromyography. In one study of 7 patients (6 end-to-end repairs and 1 neurolysis), 4 were rated as very satisfied with excellent results, whereas the remaining 3 were satisfied with good results.[4] All 7 regained symmetric motor strength when compared to the opposite side, although 3 patients had symptoms after lifting heavy objects or strenuous overhead activity. All patients underwent nerve exploration and repair between 3 and 14 months after injury. In another study of 20 patients undergoing nerve surgery, 16 had good-excellent results, whereas 4 had poor results.[2]

Thus, the early diagnosis of injury to the spinal accessory nerve is key to successful treatment. Misdiagnosis is common, and any history of significant injury and especially prior neck surgery should raise one's clinical suspicion for trapezius palsy. Based on the literature, early exploration and nerve surgery is indicated between 3 and 20 months after the injury. Persistent symptoms in active patients greater than 20 months after their injury, or with evidence of muscle fibrosis should indicate an Eden-Lange triple muscle transfer. As these are rare injuries and procedures, any surgeon undertaking a nerve exploration of the posterior cervical triangle or a complex muscle reconstruction should have precise anatomical knowledge and clinical experience with microsurgical nerve repair and muscle transfer operations.

References

1. Bigliani LU, Compito CA, Duralde XA, Wolfe IN. Transfer of the levator scapulae, rhomboid major, and rhomboid minor for paralysis of the trapezius. *J Bone Joint Surg Am.* 1996;78A:1534-1540.
2. Teboul F, Bizot P, Kakkar R, Sedel L. Surgical management of trapezius palsy. *J Bone Joint Surg Am.* 2004; 86A:1884-1890.
3. Dewar FP, Harris RI. Restoration of function of the shoulder following paralysis of the trapezius by fascial sling fixation and transplantation of the levator scapulae. *Ann Surg.* 1950;132:1111-1115.
4. Nakamichi K, Tachibana S. Iatrogenic injury to the spinal accessory nerve. Results of repair. *J Bone Joint Surg Am.* 1998;80A:1616-1621.

WHAT IS THE BEST ARTHROPLASTY OPTION IN A SHOULDER WITH RHEUMATOID ARTHRITIS?

Matthew D. Williams, MD
T. Bradley Edwards, MD

Rheumatoid arthritis is an inflammatory disease of the synovium that causes synovial hyperplasia and disabling erosive arthritis. Progression of the disease involves the entire glenohumeral joint and surrounding structures, including the bone, acromioclavicular joint, subacromial bursa, and rotator cuff tendons. The treatment algorithm for rheumatoid arthritis of the glenohumeral joint involves both nonoperative and minimally invasive arthroscopic procedures. Failure of these modalities or advanced disease at presentation may necessitate glenohumeral joint replacement to alleviate pain and improve function in these patients. Joint replacement procedures in the shoulder include hemiarthroplasty, total shoulder arthroplasty (TSA), and reverse shoulder arthroplasty. The decision about which implant is best for the treatment of rheumatoid arthritis in the shoulder is based on the progression of disease in each individual patient (ie, what anatomic structures are involved that will affect postoperative shoulder function).

Early complaints in rheumatoid patients are pain, swelling, and decreasing shoulder motion. Pain and restriction of mobility worsen with advancement of the disease. Medial migration of the humeral head causes erosion of the glenoid and obliteration of the joint space, which are visible on radiographs. Rheumatoid patients have osteopenic bone with periarticular cyst formation. These periarticular erosions affect the superior humeral head and may also be found in the glenoid. Cysts in the superior humeral head coupled with rheumatoid rotator cuff tendon degeneration lead to rotator cuff compromise. Cysts in the glenoid hasten the loss of bone stock.

Rheumatoid arthritis patients are evaluated thoroughly because in our experience they have numerous confounding concomitant problems. Importantly, radiculopathy or myelopathy secondary to cervical spine involvement causing pain or weakness must be examined. Imaging is fundamental to appropriate treatment of this group of patients. Periarticular cysts in the humeral head may affect component fixation, and rotator cuff deficiency or glenoid bone loss may preclude placement of a glenoid component altogether. Preoperative planning for shoulder arthroplasty in patients with rheumatoid arthritis includes a computed tomography (CT) arthrogram in our practice to adequately evaluate the rotator cuff and both the humeral and glenoid bone stock.

Shoulder arthroplasty in patients with advanced rheumatoid disease with an intact rotator cuff and mild glenoid bone loss is acceptable using either hemiarthroplasty or TSA with glenoid resurfacing. There has been a shift in opinion over the past few years as to whether hemiarthroplasty or TSA is best. Previously, experience with glenoid resurfacing was limited and many surgeons were not comfortable with implanting a glenoid component; therefore, total shoulder replacement cohorts were small, resulting in equal or lesser results than hemiarthroplasty.[1] However, with increasing experience and patient follow-up, the literature demonstrates that TSA produces superior results.[2,3] Collins and colleagues[2] reported on 61 patients treated with hemiarthroplasty or TSA for rheumatoid arthritis. Both treatment groups showed improvements in pain, motion, and function scores, but those undergoing TSA had greater improvement. In a large comparison study of over 300 patients followed for a mean of 11 years, Sperling and colleagues[3] found that TSA was the preferred procedure for rheumatoid arthritis of the shoulder with an intact rotator cuff.

Contraindications to TSA include glenoid bone loss and an incompetent rotator cuff. Large periarticular cysts involving the glenoid coupled with medial humeral head migration lead to severe loss of glenoid bone stock. Glenoid bone insufficient to accept and anchor a polyethylene component is a contraindication to TSA and a hemiarthroplasty should be chosen. Rotator cuff–deficient shoulders suffer from superior humeral migration and are not candidates for glenoid resurfacing secondary to glenoid failure.[4] These patients also function poorly after hemiarthroplasty due to anterior-superior instability. Rheumatoid patients with an incompetent rotator cuff are treated with reverse shoulder arthroplasty.[5]

In our practice, patients with rheumatoid arthritis awaiting shoulder replacement are placed into 1 of 3 treatment groups: those with an intact rotator cuff and adequate glenoid bone stock, those with an intact rotator cuff and poor glenoid bone stock, and those with cuff deficient shoulders (Figure 29-1). Patients with an intact rotator cuff and adequate glenoid bone stock on preoperative CT scanning to accommodate a polyethylene glenoid component are treated with TSA. We routinely employ press-fit humeral components; however, we are always prepared to use a cemented humeral stem when proximal humeral bone stock is lacking due to cyst formation. Resurfacing of the glenoid is performed with a cemented all-polyethylene component; we do not have a preference toward a keeled or pegged design. We perform a hemiarthroplasty if preoperative CT scanning demonstrates inadequate glenoid bone stock for placement of a glenoid component. Patients with rotator cuff–deficient shoulders are treated with a reverse shoulder arthroplasty (Figure 29-2).

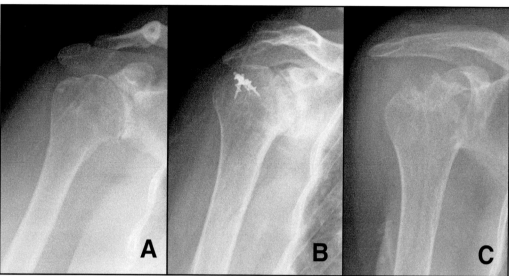

Figure 29-1. Anteroposterior shoulder radiographs of patients with rheumatoid arthritis (RA) demonstrating our stratification of patients. (A) The first x-ray portrays RA with an intact rotator cuff. (B) The second film demonstrates a cuff-deficient rheumatoid shoulder. (C) The third x-ray shows RA with both humeral head and glenoid destruction.

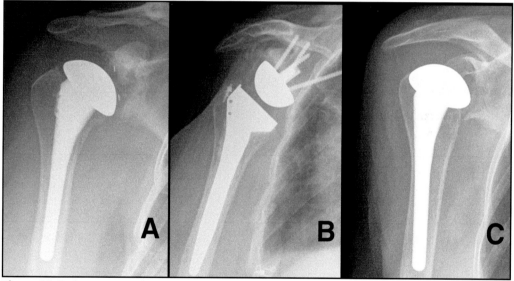

Figure 29-2. Anteroposterior postoperative radiographs demonstrating our 3 treatment options. (A) Total shoulder arthroplasty for rheumatoid shoulders with an intact rotator cuff. (B) Reverse shoulder arthroplasty for a cuff-deficient shoulder. (C) Hemiarthroplasty is reserved for rheumatoid shoulders with glenoid bone loss that does not allow glenoid component implantation.

References

1. Trail IA, Nuttall D. The results of shoulder arthroplasty in patients with rheumatoid arthritis. *J Bone Joint Surg Br.* 2002;84:1121-1125.
2. Collins DN, Harryman DT 2nd, Wirth MA. Shoulder arthroplasty for the treatment of inflammatory arthritis. *J Bone Joint Surg Am.* 2004;86:2489-2496.

3. Sperling J, Cofield RH, Schleck C. Total shoulder arthroplasty versus hemiarthroplasty for rheumatoid arthritis: results of 303 consecutive cases. Presented at the 23rd Open Meeting American Shoulder and Elbow Surgeons Specialty Day. San Diego, California, 2007.

4. Franklin JL, Barrett WP, Jackins SE, Matsen FA 3rd. Glenoid loosening in total shoulder arthroplasty: association with rotator cuff deficiency. *J Arthroplasty.* 1988;3:39-46.

5. Rittmeister M, Kerschbaumer F. Grammont reverse total shoulder arthroplasty in patients with rheumatoid arthritis and nonreconstructable rotator cuff lesions. *J Shoulder Elbow Surg.* 2001;43:2152-2159.

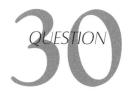

WHAT ARE THE INDICATIONS FOR A HEMIARTHROPLASTY VERSUS AN OSTEOCHONDRAL ALLOGRAFT IN A PATIENT WITH A LOCKED POSTERIOR DISLOCATION AND LARGE REVERSE HILL-SACHS LESION?

Michael Freehill, MD

There are few things that cause greater anxiety in an orthopedist's office than when a patient arrives with evidence of a chronic locked posterior dislocation. Depending on the duration of the dislocation, the humeral head defect and glenoid damage may be quite extreme. Patients with recurrent posterior dislocations, even with proper reduction, can also present with large bony defects. Surgical intervention is indicated in the setting of large bone defects after posterior dislocation. In the case of a locked posterior dislocation with a large reverse Hill-Sachs lesion, the challenging part is to determine what surgical technique is best—hemiarthroplasty or an osteochondral allograft.

In 1997, Gerber and Lambert initially described the use of allograft reconstruction for segmental defects of the humeral head in those patients who presented with a chronically locked posterior dislocation of the shoulder. In those cases, patients had a minimum of 40% involvement of the humeral articular surface and were managed with reconstruction of the humeral head utilizing allograft from an allograft femoral head segment.[1] More recently, attention has been turned to management of large, engaging Hill-Sachs lesions in anterior instability with size-matched humeral head allografts, as described by Miniaci and colleagues.[2] Surgical complications with allograft techniques include graft collapse and/or hardware complications. There are 2 described methods of allograft fixation—countersunk cancellous lag screws within the impacted allograft wedge and use of bioabsorbable screw fixation techniques.

Figure 30-1. MRI axillary view. Perched posterior shoulder dislocation with injury to posterior glenoid.

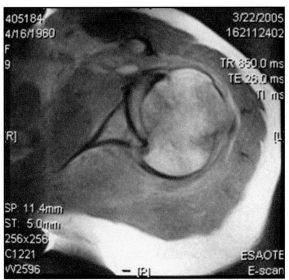

The first step in appropriately treating a chronically locked posterior dislocation is to determine the size of the humeral head defect. For defects that are 20 to 40% of the surface area of the humeral head, a modified McLaughlin procedure, which involves a transfer of the lesser tuberosity into the reverse Hill-Sachs lesion, has been described and with good success.[3] Typically, involvement of greater than 40% of the humeral head requires more aggressive surgical recommendations in the form of an arthroplasty versus an osteochondral allograft procedure. Radiographic assessment begins with an axillary view, which provides initial information regarding the estimated size of the defect and helps with the preoperative planning for the method of surgical intervention. In addition, advanced imaging of the shoulder with computed tomography (CT) or magnetic resonance imaging (MRI) scan should be obtained. This author prefers MRI imaging in order to best evaluate the glenoid articular cartilage (Figure 30-1). Severe posterior rim glenoid loss is a contra-indication for allograft reconstruction of the humeral head.

Once the size of the reverse Hill-Sachs lesion is determined, the second step in deciding what surgical technique to employ is an assessment of the patient demographics and comorbidities. With regards to age, younger patients in the absence of cardiovascular disease will likely have greater success with the allograft procedure in terms of incorporation and healing. In addition, use of the allograft in the younger patient avoids the potential complications incurred with arthroplasty in the age group. In patients aged 60 or greater with significant reverse Hill-Sachs lesions, shoulder arthroplasty is the best option. Comorbidities including significant cardiovascular disease, morbid obesity, and diabetes are more amenable to arthroplasty as the definitive treatment choice; allograft reconstruction in this population is fraught with complications, including infection, poor healing, and increased reoperation rate.

Overall management of a locked posterior dislocation with concomitant large reverse Hill-Sachs lesions can be a very challenging problem. A full medical history in combination with detailed imaging studies will help the orthopedic surgeon to determine the

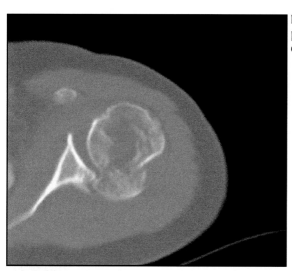

Figure 30-2. CT scan axillary view. Locked posterior shoulder dislocation, assessment of 40% injury to humeral head.

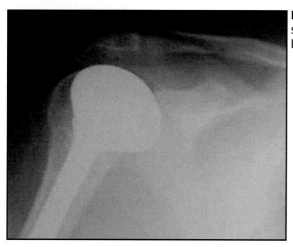

Figure 30-3. AP view. Hemiarthroplasty status post locked posterior shoulder dislocation.

appropriate treatment option. A sized-match humeral head osteochondral allograft in the young patient appears to be a very viable treatment option in cases involving greater than 40% of the humeral head surface (Figure 30-2). In patients over the age of 60 or those who have significant medical comorbidities, a hemiarthroplasty (or with severe glenoid articular surface loss, a total shoulder arthroplasty) is our procedure of choice (Figure 30-3). If an arthroplasty procedure is chosen, care must be taken to obtain proper soft-tissue balancing of the posterior capsular structures to avoid recurrent posterior instability. In addition, the implant should be placed in 15 to 20 degrees of retroversion to avoid potential recurrent posterior instability. Fixation techniques for the allograft procedure are based on surgeon preference and can include either countersunk cancellous lag screws or bioabsorbable screw fixation.

References

1. Gerber C, Lambert SM. Allograft reconstruction of segmental defects of the humeral head for the treatment of chronic locked posterior dislocation of the shoulder. *Bone Joint Surg Am.* 1996; 78:376-382.
2. Miniaci A, Hand C, Berlet G. Segmental humeral head allografts for recurrent anterior instability of the shoulder with large Hill-Sachs defects: a two to eight year follow-up. Presented at the 20th Annual Closed Meeting of the American Shoulder and Elbow Surgeons; October 10, 2003; Dana Point, CA.
3. DeZuckerman J. McLaughlin procedure for acute and chronic posterior dislocations. In: Gregg E, ed. *Master Technique in Orthopaedic Surgery: The Shoulder.* 2nd ed. Philadelphia: Lippencott Williams &Wilkins; 2004: 289-305.

What Is the Management of Symptomatic Subscapularis Deficiency After Previous Shoulder Surgery?

Gregory P. Nicholson, MD

Subscapularis deficiency after previous shoulder surgery can present in a very subtle fashion with weakness of shoulder function away from the body position or above horizontal. Most patients are not frankly unstable from subscapularis deficiency but present more with poor function and a feeling of weakness.[1-3] The two most common clinical scenarios where subscapularis deficiency would present itself are those where the subscapularis needs to be incised, reflected medially, and then re-repaired. This would include an open instability repair or shoulder arthroplasty.

A good physical examination is imperative, along with obtaining the operative note. It is important to examine for passive range of motion and active range of motion. An extensive amount of external rotation at the side as compared to the nonoperative arm is consistent with subscapularis deficiency (Figure 31-1). The belly-press sign and the lift-off test evaluate for the upper and lower subscapularis, respectively. Weakness of belly press or the inability to just hold the palm of the hand onto the abdomen (the belly-off sign[4]) can be consistent with subscapularis deficiency. This test could be done by asking the patient to hold the hand with a flat wrist onto his abdomen. If the hand comes off the belly or the elbow falls back significantly, this again is significant for subscapularis deficiency (Figure 31-2). Many patients cannot do a lift-off test because they have pain in an operative shoulder, which is not functioning well. These tests help determine if the subscapularis is functioning. It is important to test for the strength of the supraspinatus, the infraspinatus, the teres minor, the deltoid, and the scapular rotators.

If there is an arthroplasty in place, an magnetic resonance imaging (MRI) can be a very difficult study to interpret because of the artifact from the MRI. Thus, with an arthroplasty in place, I would recommend an arthrogram computed tomography (CT) scan to evaluate the status of the tendon and the muscle belly. Ultrasound is also a useful modality, but is technique and operator dependent.

Figure 31-1. An intraoperative photo demonstrating greater than 90 degrees of external rotation in a right shoulder after previous surgery. The subscapularis was torn.

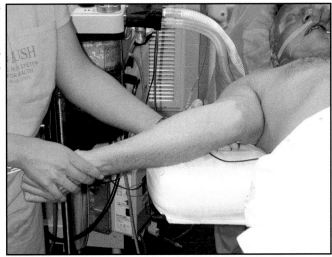

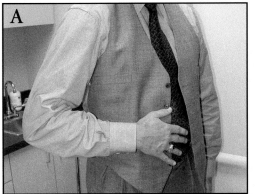

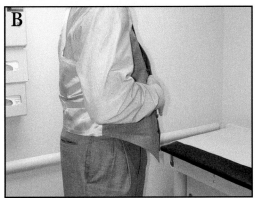

Figure 31-2. (A) The belly-press test, with the attempt to keep the elbow at the level of the front of the body. (B) The elbow has fallen back to the midaxillary line, signifying deficiency of, or poor function or, the subscapularis.

Without an arthroplasty in place, a gadolinium arthrogram MRI is an excellent study to accomplish the same things that the arthrogram CT scan did in an arthroplasty setting. If the subscapularis deficiency is discovered early after the original surgery, then re-exploration and re-repair of the subscapularis can be performed primarily. The subscapularis muscle tendon unit needs to be mobilized off the coracoid base and off the anterior glenoid rim. Importantly, it needs to be freed from the inferior capsule, which is where the axillary nerve crosses the inferior margin of the subscapularis. Thus, it is very important to identify the axillary nerve in this exploration as the subscapularis tendon is released from the inferior capsule.

The anterior capsular structures can be deficient. Thus, any time a subscapularis deficient shoulder is reoperated after previous surgery, I would recommend having allograft tendon available. This can be used to reconstruct the anterior capsule, creating an anterior capsular structure to center and prevent subluxation of the humeral head. This also allows collagen material on which to place the subscapularis repair down.

I also recommend very heavy suture in a locking type of stitch configuration such as a Krakow locking stitch and utilizing no. 5 sutures. I then bring these through the medial border of the lesser tuberosity and out the biceps groove so that there is very robust suture material woven into the subscapularis tendon and then very firm transosseous fixation. This surgery can all be done through a deltopectoral incision.

In the case of an arthroplasty with subscapularis deficiency, the same operative strategies apply. In this case, certainly an allograft tendon needs to be considered because of the previous surgery, which is much more anatomy altering, and the fact that there is a prosthetic humeral head and not a native humeral head and bone may create issues in the anterior aspect of the shoulder. In these cases, an Achilles tendon allograft can be fixed to the anterior/inferior glenoid with screws without any damage to an existing glenoid component. Then the Achilles tendon allograft can be run across to the humerus and placed through drill holes in the lesser tuberosity and then brought back across and fixated to the glenoid and/or the coracoid base.

If the subscapularis muscle tendon unit is now identifiable and can be mobilized, it can be repaired as previously discussed back to the lesser tuberosity.

If, however, the subscapularis is so deficient that it is unable to be repaired, then consideration for some type of muscle tendon transfer to substitute for the subscapularis needs to be considered. The most useful transfer is a pectoralis major transfer.[5] It will provide an adequate alternative for the action of the subscapularis in most patients, but it is not normal. This is an advanced surgery and will not fully substitute for the action of the subscapularis, and this needs to be discussed with the patient preoperatively.

Summary

The 2 most common clinical postsurgical scenarios for subscapularis deficiency are open instability repair and shoulder arthroplasty. Arthrogram CT scan is an excellent imaging study for arthroplasty issues. Gadolinium arthrogram MRI is an excellent study in the instability etiology. If the subscapularis deficiency is recognized early after the original surgery, then primary repair can be undertaken. If the subscapularis deficiency is discovered at a later date, after 4 to 6 months, and there is anterior capsular deficiency, the surgeon needs to be prepared to do a capsular reconstruction of either autograft or allograft material. In rare instances, the subscapularis is so deficient that pectoralis major transfer needs to be considered.

References

1. Miller BS, Joseph TA, Noonan TJ, et al. Rupture of the subscapsularis tendon after shoulder arthroplasty: diagnosis, treatment, and outcome. *J Shoulder Elbow Surg.* 2005;14:492-496.
2. Miller SJ, Hazrati Y, Klepps S, Chiang A, Flatow EL. Loss of subscapularis function after total shoulder replacement: a seldom recognized problem. *J Shoulder Elbow Surg.* 2003;12:29-34.
3. Scheibel M, Tsynman A, Magosch P, Schroeder RJ, Habermeyer P. Postoperative subscapularis muscle insufficiency after primary and revision open shoulder stabilization. *Am J Sports Med.* 2006;34:1586-1593.
4. Scheibel M, Magosch P, Pritsch M, Lichtenberg S, Habermeyer P. The belly-off sign: a new clinical diagnostic sign for subscapularis lesions. *Arthroscopy.* 2005;21:1229-1235.
5. Resch H, Povacz P, Ritter E, Matschi W. Transfer of the pectoralis major muscle for the treatment of irreparable rupture of the subscapularis tendon. *J Bone Joint Surg.* 2000;82A:372-382.

SECTION VII

ROTATOR CUFF QUESTIONS

When Is It Appropriate to Begin Resistive Strengthening Exercises After the Repair of a 3.5-cm Supraspinatus Tear?

R. Michael Gross, MD
Joseph Carney, MD

Rotator cuff repair rehabilitation can be most easily thought of as 3 periods of 6 weeks each. The first 6 weeks should focus on healing of the tendon. The second 6 weeks focuses on gaining full range of motion (ROM) with proper shoulder mechanics. The third 6 weeks focuses on regaining power and endurance.

During the first set of 6 weeks, it's fairly easy to notice the "quick healers," individuals who have almost keloid-like healing tendency for their tendons, as well as those with pain intolerance. Both of these groups of individuals are high risk for developing postoperative stiffness, "captured shoulder," and an unsatisfactory result. We suggest that they need an early referral to a therapist that you are familiar with and trust. They can begin closely supervised supine passive and active assisted exercises.

Most individuals don't fall into the "quick healer" category and should be relegated to home pendulum exercises, and if the tear does not involve the external rotator muscles, we feel that it is safe to begin early, active assistive external rotation of the affected extremity, with emphasis on keeping the elbow close to the body. We frequently ask the patient to put a magazine under the arm while performing this exercise. If the magazine falls, the elbow is too far away from the side. While doing both of these exercises, the patient is also asked to shrug and protract the shoulder blades. At the end of the first 6-week period, an individual should have fair comfort, good flexibility, and a reasonably good ROM.

The second 6-week period focuses on gaining full motion with normal shoulder mechanics. It is critical that the patient focuses on keeping the shoulder down while working on ROM in an effort to avoid substitution with the scapula. We find it helpful to do these exercises in front of a mirror. The exercise that we suggest is called "the punch." The

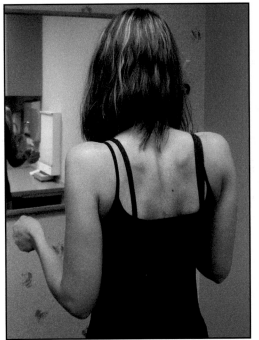

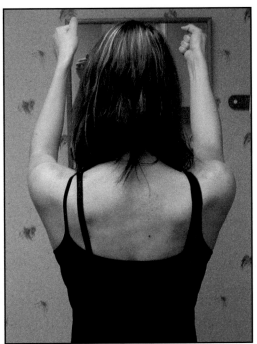

Figure 32-1. The "punch" exercise is initiated with the elbows bent 90 degrees and the arms at the side. The hands are made into light fists. The patient stations him-/herself in front of a mirror to monitor scapula substitution. The forearms are held parallel to the floor with a clenched fist. Note that the scapulas are protracted. It is difficult to over-rotate a scapula when it is held in a protracted position. The arms are then slowly elevated trying to keep the scapulas protracted and the shoulders level.

Figure 32-2. The "punch" exercise ends with the arms at shoulder height. Watching in the mirror helps prevent the scapula from "hiking up" and allowing better mechanics to the exercise.

patient watches him-/herself in a mirror. The elbows are kept close to the body and flexed at 90 degrees while the hands are held in a fist (Figure 32-1). While watching the mirror, the patient slowly punches both arms forward and holds the shoulders level (Figure 32-2). If the shoulder elevates, the punch stops, and the exercise is done again. This exercise emphasizes mobility with proper mechanics and no scapular substitution. Those who have reasonable motion and mechanics at 8 weeks can start gentle progressive internal and external rotation exercises using a Thera-Band (Hygenic Corp, Akron, OH) (again, this is assuming that the external rotator muscles are not involved in the tear). At the end of this rehabilitation segment, your patient should have close to full ROM with good shoulder mechanics.

The third set of 6 weeks focuses on power and endurance. We tend to agree with most authors in that resistive strengthening exercises should not begin until 3 months after surgery if the patient has progressed adequately and met all goals of the rehabilitation protocol on time. This allows adequate time for more complete remodeling of the tendon bone interface so as to optimize tensile strength of the repaired tendon at time of initiation of resistance activity.

Institution of resistive strengthening before tendon healing has occurred is a common cause of rotator cuff repair failure.[1]

It cannot be overemphasized that although the tendon may be strong at 12 weeks, if the mechanics are poor, the shoulder remains at risk. We view poor mechanics like a horse kicking at a stall door. It may take the horse a while but with persistence, the stall door will fall. The same can be expected from exercising a shoulder in the face of poor shoulder mechanics—with time, the rotator cuff will fail. We are frequently asked by our patients: "How do I know when I'm doing too much?" Our response is that gaining power and endurance is a job and it may be uncomfortable and on occasion miserable, but discomfort should not persist for an hour or two after the exercises. If the patient finds himself going to bed in the evening and the shoulder is more uncomfortable than it was when he got up in the morning, then that is like a runner getting ready for a marathon but overshooting his mark and developing shin splints.

Summarize

When approaching the rehabilitation of a patient with a supraspinatus repair, it is important to educate the patient that rotator cuff rehabilitation is a prolonged process. Many factors affect the course and progression of the rehabilitation protocol. Advancing too quickly can jeopardize the result of the procedure, as can ending rehabilitation prematurely. Although initiation of resistive strengthening is most often begun 3 months after surgery, it is necessary to individualize this decision to the patient and his or her rotator cuff repair, with emphasis on ROM and proper mechanics, before resistive strengthening is started.

Reference

1. Nevaiser RJ, Nevaiser TJ. Re-operation for failed rotator cuff repair: analysis of fifty cases. *J Shoulder Elbow Surg.* 1992:1:283-286.

33

WHAT ARE THE INDICATIONS FOR AN ARTHROSCOPIC SUBACROMIAL DECOMPRESSION IN A WEEKEND ATHLETE WITH SHOULDER PAIN?

Joseph Carney, MD
R. Michael Gross, MD

Impingement can be an isolated problem however, more often it is a secondary problem that is a manifestation of a more core problem such as instability or a rotator cuff tear. An isolated subacromial decompression performed on a patient who has a secondary impingement is likely to fail. This chapter deals with focuses on those individuals who have isolated subacromial impingement.

Most patients who have a shoulder impingement problem eventually recover with nonoperative intervention.[1] Successful nonoperative treatment requires breaking the cycle of inflammation and pain. The tools available to the treating physician are activity modification, anti-inflammatory medication (oral and/or injectable), and rotator cuff strength training. The goal of treatment is the same as if a door is tight in the door jam; we attempt to "dehumidify" the bursa and tendons by drawing the inflammation out of the tissue with activity modification, strengthening, and medications. There is no gold standard to accomplish this goal.

In some circumstances, it is considered more "urgent" for the patient to recover quickly in order to return to his or her sport, or there may be economic pressures for the patient that demand a more aggressive approach. In these circumstances, early referral to physical therapy for strengthening and passive modalities, as well as an early bursal injection of cortisone and anti-inflammatory medications, might be the most appropriate approach. In others, time may not be an issue and circumstances might dictate a slower, home-directed physical therapy approach. The pathway is chosen by the patient, but in either case, there are some guidelines that would could improve success.

Nonsteroidal anti-inflammatory drugs (NSAIDs) should be taken on a scheduled basis if not contraindicated by any patient comorbidities. Using NSAIDs on an as-needed basis does not allow the patient to receive the maximum benefit from the medication. A useful adjunct to the medical treatment of impingement is a course of physical therapy for passive modalities and rotator cuff strengthening. Whether the physical therapy is formal or a strict "do it yourself" protocol, it is important to structure the approach with specific benchmarks. The purpose of the physical therapy is two-fold: (1) strengthen the rotator cuff emphasizing appropriate shoulder mechanics, and (2) employ passive modalities that may help draw the inflammation out of the soft tissue.

We feel that dignified care would dictate that all non-operative treatment modalities be exhausted before surgery is considered. It is our opinion that the "price of admission" for a trip to the operating room is at least one trial of a subacromial injection of corticosteroids. If this fails, then surgery could be considered. Now let us share our thoughts on what *failure* means. If one injects an individual with a corticosteroid and the patient experiences remarkable improvement that wears off, *but not completely*, it could be considered a "step towards wellness." Under these circumstances, it would be reasonable to repeat the injection in 6 weeks and possibly a third time in another 6 weeks if, on each occasion, the patient takes a noticeable and significant step towards his or her goal of comfort and function.

Suggested durations of nonoperative treatment for subacromial impingement vary. Historically, an average of 12 months was thought to be necessary, but with newer, less invasive arthroscopic decompression techniques, the morbidity of surgical treatment has decreased suggesting that a shorter period of non-operative treatment may be appropriate before operative intervention is attempted.[2] If the patient's symptoms show unsatisfactory improvement, despite exhausting nonoperative modalities, we feel it is reasonable to explore surgical options as early as 3 months after initiation of nonoperative treatment. Regardless of the timing of surgery, the potential for success is best if the patient has achieved near symmetric range of motion and good strength of the shoulder prior to surgical intervention.

Summary

There is no true gold standard approach for deciding when a "weekend athlete" should undergo a subacromial decompression. Decompression alone can be considered when it is certain there is no other primary shoulder pathology and after nonoperative therapy has failed. An excellent preoperative response to a subacromial injection usually bodes well for surgical decompression success. We do not subscribe to a set interval of non-operative care. We do feel that a trial of at least one cortisone injection, oral anti-inflammatory medications, and a legitimate effort by a qualified physical therapist should be attempted before surgery is suggested. Given that position, it would be difficult to appropriately cover all of these bases in less than 3 months.

References

1. Bigliani LU. Levine WN. Subacromial impingement syndrome. *J Bone Joint Surg Am*. 1997;79:1854-1868.
2. Norlin R. Arthroscopic subacromial decompression versus open acromioplasty. *Arthroscopy*. 1989;5:321-323.

A 35-YEAR-OLD HAS SUBACROMIAL IMPINGEMENT SYMPTOMS. AT ARTHROSCOPY, A HYPERMOBILE MESO-ACROMIALE— UNFUSED ACROMIAL EPIPHYSIS—WAS FOUND. HOW DO YOU MANAGE A PATIENT WITH A SYMPTOMATIC OS ACROMIALE (MESO-ACROMION) THAT IS DUE TO AN UNFUSED ACROMIAL EPIPHYSIS?

Sumant G. "Butch" Krishnan, MD
Paul Jarman, MD

The OS acromiale results from a failure of fusion of the acromial apophysis of the scapula and occurs in nearly 8% of the population (Figure 34-1). Normally, 4 centers (the pre-, meso, meta-, and basi-acromion) fuse to form the acromion. The centers appear at around age 15 and should have completed their union to the scapula by the age of 22 to 25 years. The most common anomaly is the failure of the meso-acromion to fuse to the meta-acromion, and it may cause symptoms through inflammation of the synchondrosis, mechanical subacromial impingement by the mobile fragment from downward pull of the deltoid, or coexistent cuff pathology.[1-3]

For us, the appropriate management of this lesion (even if discovered intraoperatively) is dependent on the preoperative history and examination. We try to determine if the primary source of pain is subacromial impingement or the mobile synchondrosis.

Figure 34-1. Axillary view demonstrating a meso-acromial fragment.

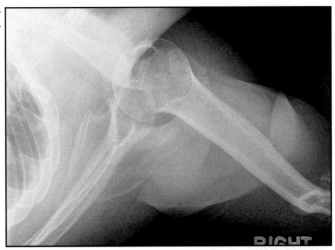

Impingement tests (Neer's Sign) may be positive and/or palpation of the fragment may induce either local pain or impingement symptoms due to a mobile fragment pressing on the underlying cuff.[2,4] We make the diagnostic distinction via injection of local anesthetic into the subacromial space. If this test eradicates all of the patient's pain with impingement tests, we suspect pain from subacromial impingement and not from the mobile synchondrosis. If it does not, this may be suggestive of a symptomatic OS acromiale. A further injection may be administered to the synchondrosis itself. This may relieve up to 100% of the patient's typical pain. Radiologically, the lesion is best appreciated on the axillary lateral film. On the anteroposterior (AP) film, there may be the appearance of a double shadow at the acromion indicating the OS. If a magnetic resonance imaging (MRI) scan is performed, it will demonstrate the OS acromiale, and may demonstrate edema at the junction of the OS fragment and the anterior acromion in pathologic cases. To confirm the diagnosis of a symptomatic OS, we perform a technetium bone scan. Increased uptake in the synchondrosis leads to the definitive diagnosis of a symptomatic OS.

As stated previously, our preferred operative technique is determined by the preoperative assessment. If the OS acromiale is not deemed to be symptomatic and the reason for the procedure is impingement rather than synchondrotic pain, the lesion may be debrided. Our preferred technique is to shell out the fragment to the cortical rim. This limits the potential for future impingement on the rotator cuff, but does not compromise the deltoid attachment. If the acromioclavicular joint is to be debrided, care must be taken with the clavicular debridement, as excessive bony resection may destabilize the deltoid attachment. Often, treatment of the OS is sufficient to decompress this joint as well.

If the OS acromiale is symptomatic and demonstrates increased uptake on bone scan preoperatively, we favor an open approach for either excision of the entire OS or fixation of the symptomatic fragment. Excision and deltoid reattachment may result in significant deltoid dysfunction, and we therefore reserve this technique for smaller fragments (preacromial fragments) or as a salvage after failed internal fixation. Because of the potential difficulty obtaining union after reduction and fixation of a symptomatic OS fragment, we prefer to provide both mechanical compression and biological augmentation (Figure 34-2). The synchondrosis is debrided with a motorized burr, reduced, and grafted

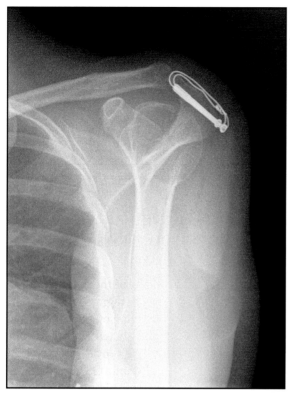

Figure 34-2. Fixation with cannulated screws and tension-band wire supplementation.

with a tricortical bone wedge from the scapular spine. Compression across the fragment is provided by 2 cannulated lag screws, supplemented by tension-band wire passed through the cannulated screw. This lower profile construct (when compared with other reported techniques) may lead to less symptomatic hardware in the postoperative setting.[1-4] Attention must be paid to the handling of the deltoid, which we prefer to split rather than completely detach to avoid violation of the acromial branches of the thoracoacromial artery. Care must be taken to insure that hardware does not invade the subacromial space and, at the completion of the procedure, the deltoid attachment must be secure.

References

1. Peckett WRC, Gunther SB, Harper GD, et al. Internal fixation of symptomatic OS acromiale: a series of twenty-six cases. *J Shoulder Elbow Surg.* 2004:13:381-385.
2. Pagnani MJ, Mathis CE, Salman CG. Painful OS acromiale (or unfused acromial apophysis) in athletes. *J Shoulder Elbow Surg.* 2006;15:432-435.
3. Ortiguera CJ, Buss DD. Surgical management of the symptomatic OS acromiale. *J Shoulder Elbow Surg.* 2002; 11:521-528.
4. Abboud JA, Silverberg D, Pepe M, et al. Surgical treatment of OS acromiale with and without associated rotator cuff tears. *J Shoulder Elbow Surg.* 2006;15:265-270.

35

WHAT ARE THE INDICATIONS FOR LONG HEAD OF BICEPS TENODESIS VERSUS TENOTOMY IN A PATIENT UNDERGOING ROTATOR CUFF REPAIR?

Clifford G. Rios, MD
Robert A. Arciero, MD
Anthony A. Romeo, MD
Augustus D. Mazzocca, MD

Proximal biceps pathology is frequently associated with rotator cuff disease, and infrequently an isolated entity, but identifying diagnoses concomitantly can be difficult. We rely on a combination of history and physical examination findings to recognize patients with biceps involvement. First, these patients may complain of anterior shoulder pain rather than, or in addition to, lateral arm pain characteristic of isolated rotator cuff tears. On examination, tenderness in the anterior shoulder over the bicipital groove that radiates distally into the biceps muscle is characteristic. This point of tenderness should move laterally as the arm is externally rotated. We find Yergason's test helpful in the setting of proximal biceps instability. Another test we use is the subpectoral biceps tendon test. For this test, we palpate the biceps tendon in the axilla, where it is found beneath the pectoralis major tendon, during resisted internal rotation of the arm. Tenderness here suggests pathology of the biceps tendon. This maneuver may produce discomfort in a normal shoulder, so it is important to compare the side in question to the unaffected side. Pain greater on the affected side, which is alleviated by intra-articular injection of lidocaine, suggests pathology in the bicipital groove (ie, positive subpectoral biceps tendon test). The tendon sheath of the long head of the biceps is continuous with the glenohumeral joint and explains how intra-articular administration of lidocaine can relieve symptoms attributable to this tendon.

Significant proximal biceps pathology can be confirmed by arthroscopic examination. With a probe in the anterior portal, we pull the biceps tendon into the glenohumeral joint to evaluate the tendon's mobility and structural lesions. Because biceps tendon pathology is most often in the intertubercular groove portion, it is critical that you draw this part of the tendon into the joint. This pathology can range from fraying to complete rupture as well as dislocation from the intertubercular groove. It is unknown how much biceps fraying is associated with structural change; however, some authors have proposed 30% to 50%. We do not use a particular percent of fraying as indication for addressing the biceps tendon concomitantly with rotator cuff repair. Rather, we use the myriad findings in the history and physical examination that suggest proximal biceps pathology as our indication to treat this tendon. If these examination findings suggest proximal biceps tendon pathology, we will perform a biceps tenotomy or tenodesis. Attempts at stabilizing the biceps tendon have resulted in a secondary rupture of the tendon in at least 25% of the cases in one series, and have been associated with stiffness or loss of external rotation due to fixation of the biceps within the bicipital groove.[1] Therefore, we also treat instability of the biceps tendon with a tenotomy or tenodesis, rather than attempting reconstruction of the coracohumeral ligament attachment on the humerus.

We decide between biceps tenotomy and tenodesis on a case-by-case basis. In fact, we will always let the patient decide after discussing the advantages and disadvantages of each technique. Age is not an independent predictor of whether we perform a biceps tenodesis or tenotomy. The issues we address include deformity, weakness in flexion and supination, and muscle belly discomfort or cramping. Depending on the shape and girth of the patient's arm, there may or may not be a palpable defect. In a recent review by Boileau and colleagues, 72 patients with irreparable rotator cuff tears were treated with either biceps tenotomy (39 cases) or tenodesis (33 cases).[2] Biceps tenotomy and tenodesis both were effective in alleviating pain in elderly patients with irreparable rotator cuff tears associated with a lesion. Only 16 patients noticed a "Popeye" sign and none of them were bothered by it. Another review of 160 patients with a mean age of 54 and 58 years (80 with biceps tenodesis, 80 with tenotomy) showed no difference among groups in the grade of muscle spasms or cosmetic appearance of the arm.[3] Other authors have found no deformity following this biceps tenotomy.

It has been reported in the literature that 20% of forearm supination strength and 8% to 20% of elbow flexion strength are lost following spontaneous proximal biceps rupture. Recently, Maynou and colleagues found that after biceps tenotomy in patients with a massive, irreparable cuff tear, muscle force for elbow flexion-supination was decreased by 40% compared with that in an age-, gender-, and dominance-matched control group.[4] In the nonlaborer, nonathlete, especially in the nondominant arm, most patients do not notice this strength deficit during their routine activities. These patients will likely do well with tenotomy. We also lean toward tenotomy in patients with medical comorbidities such as diabetes or obesity as well. Conversely, a patient who is more muscular or whose activities are more physically demanding may benefit from biceps tenodesis.

If we proceed with tenodesis, we perform a subpectoral biceps tenodesis[5] (Figures 35-1 to 35-4). We do not incorporate the biceps into the rotator cuff repair for 2 reasons. Firstly, it leaves the tendon within the intertubercular groove, which may be a cause of persistent pain. Secondly, the incorporated biceps tendon can place tension on the rotator cuff repair, which is detrimental to cuff healing.

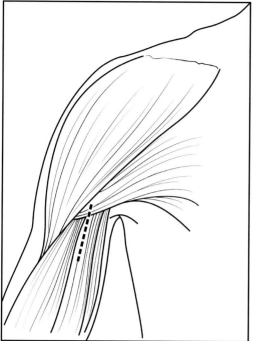

Figure 35-1. After completing an arthroscopic tenotomy, we make the skin incision for the subpectoral open biceps tenodesis in the medial one third of the arm, extending 1 cm superior to the inferior border of the pectoralis tendon to 3 cm below this border. This tendon can be palpated by resisted internal rotation with the arm abducted and internally rotated 10 to 15 degrees. (Reprinted with permission from Mazzocca AD, Rios CG, Romeo AA, Arciero RA. Subpectoral biceps tenodesis with interference screw fixation. *Arthroscopy.* 2005;21(7):896.e1-7.)

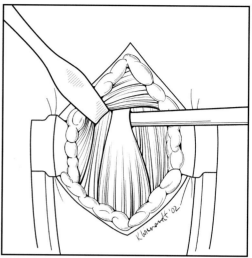

Figure 35-2. Locate the biceps tendon in the medial third of the arm by dissecting through the superficial fascia and then using blunt dissection to palpate the tendon. Retract the pectoralis deltoid complex superiorly with a Hohmann retractor. If needed, you may place a blunt Chandler retractor on the medial side of the humerus to retract the coracobrachialis and short head of the biceps. Be careful, as vigorous medial retraction may injure the musculocutaneous nerve. (Reprinted with permission from Mazzocca AD, Rios CG, Romeo AA, Arciero RA. Subpectoral biceps tenodesis with interference screw fixation. *Arthroscopy.* 2005;21(7):896.e1-7.)

Postoperative activity is typically dictated by the procedures that have been performed in conjunction with the biceps tenodesis or tenotomy. With a rotator cuff repair, passive range of motion (ROM) of the shoulder is indicated for the first 6 weeks, followed by a gradual progression from active-assisted ROM to active motion. Elbow ROM and grip strengthening can progress as tolerated without concern for the biceps tenodesis. Strengthening exercises are typically held until 6 weeks after the surgical procedure. In the case of cuff debridement and biceps tenodesis, this represents a conservative rehabilitation protocol; it may be modified to allow earlier motion if needed, such that many tenodesis patients can resume activity as tolerated at week 2, but they are informed of the risks.

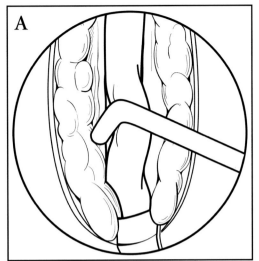

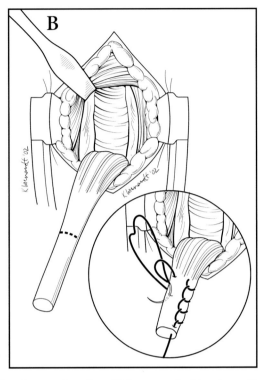

Figure 35-3. (A) Use a probe to withdraw the tendon from the joint and out of the incision. (B) To ensure appropriate tensioning, we excise 20 mm of the diseased portion of the tendon. The musculotendinous border of the biceps muscle should lie directly under the inferior edge of the pectoralis tendon. We place a Krakow or other type of interrupted tendon or whipstitch in the 10 to 15 mm of tendon proximal to the musculotendonous junction. This amount of tendon will be placed into the bone tunnel, allowing the musculotendonous junction to rest in its exact anatomical location underneath the inferior border of the pectoralis major tendon. (Reprinted with permission from Mazzocca AD, Rios CG, Romeo AA, Arciero RA. Subpectoral biceps tenodesis with interference screw fixation. *Arthroscopy.* 2005;21(7):896.e1-7.)

Figure 35-4. We create a 7- or 8-mm bone tunnel with an acorn reamer and remove the bone debris. We place one suture through the Bio-Tenodesis driver and one suture is left out. The driver is then placed with the tendon into the hole so there is a secure fit with the driver in the tendon place into the bone tunnel. Generally the size screw used is the size of the reamer (eg, an 8-mm reamer equals an 8 by 23-mm Bio-Tenodesis screw [Arthrex, Naples, FL]). (Reprinted with permission from Mazzocca AD, Rios CG, Romeo AA, Arciero RA. Subpectoral biceps tenodesis with interference screw fixation. *Arthroscopy.* 2005;21(7):896.e1-7.)

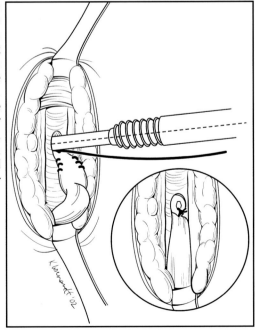

References

1. Walch G, Nové-Josserand L, Boileau P, Lévigne C. Subluxations and dislocations of the tendon of the long head of the biceps. *J Shoulder Elbow Surg.* 1998;7:100-108.
2. Boileau P, Baqué F, Valerio L, Ahrens P, Chuinard C, Trojani C. Isolated arthroscopic biceps tenotomy or tenodesis improves symptoms in patients with massive irreparable rotator cuff tears. *J Bone Joint Surg Am.* 2007;89A:747-757.
3. Osbahr DC, Diamond AB, Speer KP. The cosmetic appearance of the biceps muscle after long-head tenotomy versus tenodesis. *Arthroscopy.* 2002;18:483-487.
4. Maynou C, Mehdi N, Cassagnaud X, Audebert S, Mestdagh H. Clinical results of arthroscopic tenotomy of the long head of the biceps brachii in full thickness tears of the rotator cuff without repair: 40 cases. *Rev Chir Orthop Repar Appar Mot.* 2005;91:300-306.
5. Mazzocca AD, Rios CG, Romeo AA, Arciero RA. Subpectoral biceps tenodesis with interference screw fixation. *Arthroscopy.* 2005;21:896.

QUESTION 36

WHAT ARE THE INDICATIONS FOR DÉBRIDEMENT VERSUS REPAIR OF A PARTIAL ARTICULAR-SIDE TENDON AVULSION LESION?

Sumant G. "Butch" Krishnan, MD
John Reineck, MD

Partial articular-side tendon avulsion (PASTA) lesions of the rotator cuff were first described by Codman in 1934 as "rim-rent" tears. These tears, which are the most common partial cuff tears, begin in the hypovascular watershed zone of the cuff (usually as degenerative tears) and have been shown to have no capacity for spontaneous healing. In overhead athletes, tension overload phenomena can occur in this same area to create symptomatic partial undersurface supraspinatus tearing. When nonoperative measures fail, operative management is indicated and ranges from simple debridement to transtendon repair to takedown and repair of the cuff.[1-2]

The most important aspect of management for us, prior to surgical management, is to perform an appropriate examination and preoperative radiographic evaluation of the injured cuff. When magnetic resonance imaging (MRI) scan confirms a significant partial articular-side cuff tear (Figure 36-1), we utilize a lidocaine injection test in the subacromial space. This should anesthesize the subacromial space and relieve pain with impingement maneuvers (Neer's test). If the shoulder still demonstrates pain-free weakness with supraspinatus testing, we consider that PASTA lesion as "structurally significant" and lean toward operative repair versus simple debridement.

The appropriate surgical treatment of PASTA lesions remains controversial. Retrospective work has demonstrated that tears subjectively greater than 50% of tendon thickness (on arthroscopic examination) have poor outcomes with debridement alone.[1] However, objective measurement and determination of percentage of tendon thickness also remains difficult and variable.[2,3] Intraoperative devices have been developed to aid

Figure 36-1. Coronal oblique fat-suppressed MRI sequence demonstrating PASTA lesion.

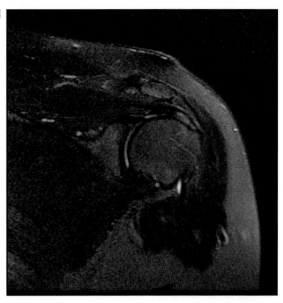

with this measurement, but controversy still exists regarding the appropriate measurement of tendon thickness and percentage torn. Based on recent anatomical descriptions of the cuff footprint, we use a modification of the Ellman classification to determine percentage of tendon torn based on bone exposed at the base of the supraspinatus footprint: if the distance between the articular margin and the remaining tendon is <3 mm, this is approximately <25% of tendon thickness; if exposed bone is <6 mm, this is <50% of the tendon; and if bone is >6 mm, this is >50% of the tendon. We feel that PASTA lesions with >6 mm of exposed bone are the structurally significant tears requiring repair.[1-3]

We also utilize the width of bone exposed on the greater tuberosity in the sagittal plane (anterior to posterior) to help determine structural significance of the PASTA lesion. If the lesion is <1 cm in width in the anteroposterior (AP) plane, this generally correlates with a structurally intact tendon and debridement only is considered. If the lesion is >1 cm AP width, this is a structurally significant tear requiring repair. Finally, based on the anatomy of the cuff and its 5 layers of thickness, we consider any cleavage of the tendon indicative of structural significance (whether identified on MRI or on arthroscopic examination). We feel that this type of cleavage indicates interstitial injury that may be structurally significant, requiring repair (Figure 36-2).

When operative repair is deemed necessary, we prefer to complete degenerative PASTA tears through the bursal surface and then repair with a double-row technique (Figure 36-3). Based on cuff anatomy, the remaining tissue on the bursal side of the cuff is not normal in these degenerative PASTA lesions and transtendon techniques may further injure that cuff. The operative success of this algorithm has been reported in the peer-reviewed literature.[3] For the overhead athlete with tension-overload phenomena and an otherwise normal tendon, we perform a transtendon repair technique to satisfy footprint restoration.

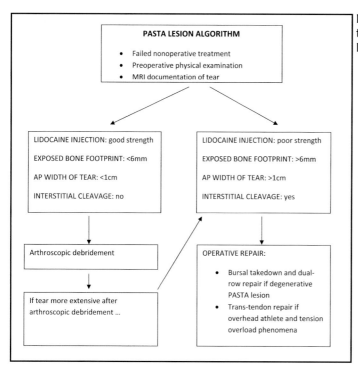

Figure 36-2. Authors' preferred treatment algorithm for PASTA lesions.

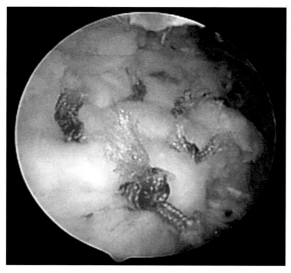

Figure 36-3. Arthroscopic view of double-row rotator cuff repair.

References

1. Weber SC. Arthroscopic debridement and acromioplasty versus mini-open repair in the management of significant partial-thickness tears of the rotator cuff. *Orthop Clin North Am.* 1997;28:79-82.
2. Wolff AB, Sethi P, Sutton KM, et al. Partial-thickness rotator cuff tears. *J Am Acad Orthop Surg.* 2006;14:715-725.
3. Deutsch A. Arthroscopic repair of partial-thickness tears of the rotator cuff. *J Shoulder Elbow Surg.* 2007;16:193-201.

WHAT ARE THE INDICATIONS TO UTILIZE A ROTATOR CUFF AUGMENTATION PATCH IN THE REPAIR OF A LARGE OR MASSIVE ROTATOR CUFF TEAR?

Matthew T. Provencher, MD, LCDR, MC, USNR
Gregory P. Nicholson, MD

One of our biggest treatment challenges is the successful, intact healing of a repair of a chronic large or massive full-thickness tear of the rotator cuff. We know in this clinical entity that the healing capacity of a chronic rotator cuff tear is diminished due to poor tissue quality and compromised blood supply. In addition, the muscle-tendon units are frequently subjected to high amounts of stress in order to afford a reasonable repair construct. Changes associated with chronic large or massive rotator cuff tears have lead to a high rate of failure after primary surgical repair and a high rate of tendon re-rupture.[1]

Tissue augmentation has long been recognized for its potential ability to improve biomechanical stability and healing in a variety of tendon and ligament repairs. Rotator cuff patches have the potential capacity to improve the healing environment, which is an attractive option given that an intact rotator cuff following repair demonstrates better functional outcomes.[1] In general, rotator cuff patches are composed of a collagenous matrix, which is derived from xenogeneic or allogeneic human tissues, depending upon manufacturer. Human sources include processed human dermal tissue, whereas animal sources include porcine small intestine submucosa (SIS), porcine dermis, and equine pericardium (Table 37-1).

Although a variety of animal and biomechanical models have shown promise of rotator cuff patches, there remains a paucity of clinical evidence to support their routine use. However, some recent evidence may support their efficacy in very early follow-up studies. The benefits of an extracellular matrix (ECM) patch are compelling and include retention of the native three-dimensional structure, with preservation of collagen, proteins, growth factors, and proteoglycans.[2]

Table 37-1

Commercially Available Rotator Cuff Patches

Product Name	Manufacturer	Licensing/Distributor	Tissue Type	Source	Sizes	Thickness	Cross-Linked/Irradiated	Other Information
GraftJacket Regenerative Tissue Matrix	LifeCell (Branchburg, NJ)	Wright Medical Technology (Arlington, TX)	Dermis	Human	5x5 cm; 5x10 cm, GraftJacket Extreme 4x7 cm	1.0 mm (Extreme 2.0 mm)	No/No	Hydration prior to use (10 to 15 mins)
BioBlanket	Kensey Nash Corporation (Exton, PA)	Not yet available					Yes/Gamma	
TissueMend	TEI Biosciences (Boston, MA)	Stryker (Mahwah, NJ)	Dermis	Bovine	5x6 cm	1.1 mm and 1.2 mm	No/No	Hydrated less than 1 minute
Zimmer Collagen Repair patch	Tissue Science Laboratories (Aldershot, Hampshire, UK)	Zimmer (Warsaw, IN)	Dermis	Porcine	5x10 cm	1.5 mm	Yes/Gamma (?)	Stored at room temperature; hydration not required
CuffPatch Bioengineered Tissue Reinforcement	Organogenesis (Canton, MA)	Arthrotek (Warsaw, IN)	SIS	Porcine	6.5x9 cm	0.6 to 1.0 mm	Yes/Gamma	Packaged hydrated; hydration not required
Restore Orthobiologic Implant	DePuy Orthopaedics (Warsaw, IN)	DePuy Orthopaedics (Warsaw, IN)	SIS	Porcine	63 mm diameter (circular)	1.0 mm	No/Electron beam	Hydration 5 to 10 minutes
OrthADAPT	Pegasus Biologics (Irvine, CA)	Pegasus Biologics	Pericardium	Equine	3x3 cm up to 9x10 cm, strips also available	0.5 mm	Yes/No	

Data on the graft characteristics, tissue origin, and tissue type are provided. (Adapted with permission from Derwin et al. Commercial extracellular matrix scaffolds for rotator cuff tendon repair. Biomechanical, biochemical, and cellular properties. *J Bone Joint Surg.* 2006;88:2665-2672.)

In an in vitro biomechanical testing model, Barber and colleagues demonstrated that the GraftJacket (157 N: thin; 229 N: extreme) had a significantly higher load to failure than CuffPatch (32 N), Restore (38 N), Zimmer Collagen Repair Patch (128 N), and TissueMend (70 to 76 N). The failure occurred by suture pullout. Overall, allograft human skin was the strongest (GraftJacket) followed by porcine (Zimmer), bovine skin (TissueMend), and SIS patches (Restore and CuffPatch). Most SIS implants demonstrate the weakest strength from 1 to 2 weeks postimplantation in a preclinical model,[2] which rapidly increases over the next 3 to 12 months. By 3 months, most studies have demonstrated that the ultimate strength of the SIS implant is similar to a reimplanted tendon.[2] In dermal interpositional grafts, the load to failure has been shown to be equivalent to control specimens by 12 weeks,[3] and remained about the same from 3 months to 6 months (increased from 539 N at 3 months to 552 N at 6 months). Other mechanical properties, such as ultimate stress, were equivalent to control groups at 6 months.

Surgical Indications and Techniques

The clinical indications for either ECM patch augmentation or interposition remain poorly defined; however, ECM patches have been described using both open and arthroscopic techniques as patch augmentation or interposition. We recommend considering the use of an ECM patch in the setting of a chronic tear in a relatively young patient who is not a candidate for alternative arthroplasty treatment (reverse shoulder, for example). This can certainly be applied to the revision rotator cuff case in which the tear is large or massive (usually greater than 4 to 5 cm, anterior to posterior), in a younger patient, that has either failed initial surgery, or who is at risk for repair failure (fatty infiltrate with some level of retraction). We do not use the patch in smaller and medium-sized tears, and also do not recommend use in large and massive tears that show minimal cuff degeneration.

We have found best results when the ECM patch is utilized in an augmentation (or onlay fashion) versus interpositional usage (using an ECM patch as an intercalary implant). We have utilized a combination of arthroscopic and open techniques to accomplish ECM patch augmentation. A double-row transosseous equivalent technique if performed followed by mini-open ECM patch augmentation provides medial row fixation, approximately 15 to 20 mm medial to the lateral edge of cuff attachment (Figure 37-1). Utilizing 2 to 3 medial anchors, the rotator cuff medial row is tied and the sutures pulled out through the anterior portal (not cut). One limb from each of the anchor sites is used for a transosseous equivalent technique,and secured to the greater tuberosity. Once tied, the suture limbs from the anchors can be utilized to achieve initial fixation of the ECM patch, with 2-0 braided polyester to fill the gaps at about 5-mm intervals. During transfer of the patch, the suture limbs from the anchors can be placed with the patch still outside the shoulder with a free needle, and the patch shuttled down the anchor suture limbs. The patch is trimmed to obtain optimal coverage (2 to 3 cm medial to the lateral edge, and approximately 1 cm lateral to the lateral tendon edge, with anterior-posterior coverage over the tear). The final shape of the patch is generally ovoid. The ECM patch is palpated and the shoulder brought through a range of motion to ensure no prominences or acromial impingement areas. The mini-open incision is closed with standard techniques. This procedure can be modified to perform an intercalary (interpositional) repair; however, we recommend that the majority of the interpositional repair be performed via open techniques.

Figure 37-1. A 47-year-old male with chronic, massive rotator cuff tear 8 months after initial repair attempt that failed. A rotator cuff ECM patch (GraftJacket) was used in an augmentation fashion with a mini-open technique. It is sutured into place using remaining suture limbs from 2 medial anchors and 3 lateral transosseous equivalent type of anchors. Additional 2-0 polyester-braided sutures are placed in simple vertical fashion to ensure no prominences and smooth tracking under the acromion.

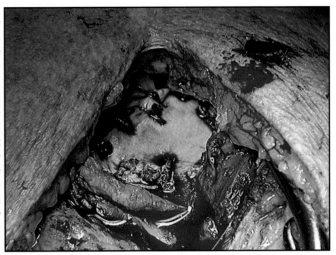

All-arthroscopic augmentation techniques have been described[4,5] and are similar to the above technique, except that the ECM patch is brought through a cannula. Suture management is critical to the success of arthroscopic procedures, and accessory portals are utilized when necessary (anterolateral, posteromedial) to "park" sutures and avoid tangling and twists. Mulberry knots have been advocated and are placed in the 4 corners of the repair to facilitate graft passage down the lateral cannula with a trocar. Additional sutures may be placed to completely secure the graft with a variety of available suture passers. Alternatively, anchors may be utilized to accomplish a 4-quadrant repair. Each limb is retrieved through the central-lateral cannula to appropriately tension and secure the graft.

The use of ECM biologic patches for the treatment of chronic, large, and massive rotator cuff tears is an emerging field. An extensive amount of basic science and preclinical models have demonstrated that an ECM patch may offer improved healing rates with a biomechanical profile that nearly reproduces the characteristics of the native rotator cuff tendon. Unfortunately, the small amount of available clinical evidence has not been as encouraging, which underscores the difficulties in extrapolating animal rotator cuff studies to human application. In addition, one should keep in mind the exact use of the ECM patch when interpreting studies—as an augmentation (onlay) versus an interpositional (intercalary) technique, which may significantly alter the overall efficacy of the ECM patch. In regards to specific patches, the small intestine submucosa (porcine derived) has shown a higher inflammatory response in the early stages, with resorption of the graft material; however, dermal grafts (both allogeneic and xenogeneic sources) also demonstrate some degree of inflammatory response, but less resorption of the graft. It remains difficult to say whether the degree of early inflammatory response is beneficial to the overall healing process. The use of ECM patches for either augmentation or intercalary repair of chronic large and massive rotator cuff tears continues to evolve; however, predictable clinical results have yet to be demonstrated.

References

1. Yamaguchi K, Ditsios K, Middleton WD, Hildebolt CF, Galatz LM, Teefey SA. The demographic and morphological features of rotator cuff disease. A comparison of asymptomatic and symptomatic shoulders. *J Bone Joint Surg Am.* 2006;88:1699-1704.
2. Zalavras CG, Gardocki R, Huang E, Stevanovic M, Hedman T, Tibone J. Reconstruction of large rotator cuff tendon defects with porcine small intestinal submucosa in an animal model. *J Shoulder Elbow Surg.* 2006; 15:224-231.
3. Adams JE, Zobitz ME, Reach JS Jr., An KN, Steinmann SP. Rotator cuff repair using an acellular dermal matrix graft: an in vivo study in a canine model. *Arthroscopy.* 2006;22:700-709.
4. Labbe MR. Arthroscopic technique for patch augmentation of rotator cuff repairs. *Arthroscopy.* 2006;22:1136 e1131-e1136.
5. Seldes RM, Abramchayev I. Arthroscopic insertion of a biologic rotator cuff tissue augmentation after rotator cuff repair. *Arthroscopy.* 2006;22:113-116.

MAGNETIC RESONANCE IMAGING SHOWS A 1-CM SUPRASPINATUS TEAR WITH 5 MM OF RETRACTION AND NO ATROPHY OF THE MUSCLE. WHAT ARE THE INDICATIONS FOR CONSERVATIVE MANAGEMENT VERSUS SURGICAL INTERVENTION IN A 55-YEAR-OLD GOLFER WITH NIGHT PAIN AND INABILITY TO PLAY GOLF?

John-Erik Bell, MD
Christopher S. Ahmad, MD

This is a common presentation in a typical orthopedic shoulder clinic. The literature does not support a "right" answer to this question, but does provide data to help in making a decision that both the surgeon and patient can feel comfortable with. It is important to understand the natural history of rotator cuff tears. In a cohort of asymptomatic volunteers age 50 to 59, 13% were found to have full-thickness rotator cuff tears by ultrasound.[1] It is not known why some full-thickness tears are symptomatic and some are not, but few surgeons would recommend surgery to an entirely asymptomatic patient based solely on an imaging study. The problem is that full-thickness rotator cuff tears have been shown to heal poorly. A thin, fibrovascular scar tissue can form between the cuff edge and the tuberosity, but is of poor biomechanical strength. In addition, more than 50% of full-thickness rotator cuff tears will progress in size over time. This progression is accompanied by scarring of the retracted tendon, with fatty infiltration and atrophy of the corresponding rotator cuff muscles, and difficulty with repair when compared to a smaller, less retracted tendon with good muscle quality.

There is ample literature discussing nonoperative treatment of full-thickness rotator cuff tears.[2-4] Overall success rates range from 25 to 82%, with pain relief ranging from 45% to 82%.[2] Although range of motion typically improved, strength did not improve with nonoperative treatment. Poor prognostic factors for nonoperative treatment include tears greater than 1 cm, preclinical symptoms greater than 1 year, severe weakness on initial presentation, and pain interrupting sleep.[4,5] Lashgari and Yamaguchi[6] divide patients with rotator cuff tears into 3 categories: Group 1 consists of those not at risk for irreversible changes in the near future, group 2 consists of those at risk for irreversible changes with prolonged nonsurgical treatment, and group 3 consists of those in whom irreversible changes have already occurred. Group 1 patients have tendonopathy or partial-thickness tears and in these patients, nonoperative treatment is unlikely to lead to irreversible changes. The patient in this question is in group 2, which includes patients with small and medium cuff tears, age under 60 years, acute tears, or recent loss of function. For these patients, we typically recommend surgical treatment due to its predictable pain relief and minimization of the chances of ultimate tear progression and further disability.

To us, it makes sense to approach symptomatic, small full-thickness tears in young, active patients such as this with a discussion regarding the advantages and disadvantages of surgical treatment. If the patient elects surgery, one must then decide on open versus arthroscopic repair. Clinical data support the assertion that arthroscopic and open rotator cuff repair techniques lead to similar clinical results.[7] The structural integrity of small and medium rotator cuff tears repaired arthroscopically seems to be better maintained over time than for large and massive tears.[8,9] In addition, arthroscopic repair minimizes deltoid injury, thereby reducing postoperative pain and adhesions, and may expedite return to activities such as golf. For these reasons, we would advocate an arthroscopic repair of the small tear in this young, active patient with a double-row suture-bridge technique. If the patient elects nonoperative treatment, we would recommend physical therapy and anti-inflammatory medication with the addition of a repeat magnetic resonance imaging (MRI) scan in approximately 4 to 6 months to assess tear progression (Figure 38-1). If tear progression is observed, we would then further advocate surgery (Figure 38-2).

References

1. Tempelhof S, Rupp S, Seil R. Age-related prevalence of rotator cuff tears in asymptomatic shoulders. *J Shoulder Elbow Surg.* 1999;8:296-299.
2. Bokor DJ, Hawkins RJ, Huckell GH, Angelo RL, Schickendantz MS. Results of nonoperative management of full-thickness tears of the rotator cuff. *Clin Orthop Relat Res.* 1993:103-110.
3. Ruotolo C, Fow JE, Nottage WM. The supraspinatus footprint: an anatomic study of the supraspinatus insertion. *Arthroscopy.* 2004;20:246-249.
4. Hawkins RH, Dunlop R. Nonoperative treatment of rotator cuff tears. *Clin Orthop Relat Res.* 1995:178-188.
5. Bartolozzi A, Andreychik D, Ahmad S. Determinants of outcome in the treatment of rotator cuff disease. *Clin Orthop Relat Res.* 1994:90-97.
6. Lashgari C, Yamaguchi K. Natural history and nonsurgical treatment of rotator cuff disorders. In: Norris TR, ed. *Orthopaedic Knowledge Update: Shoulder and Elbow 2.* Rosemont, IL: American Academy of Orthopaedic Surgeons; 2002:155-162.

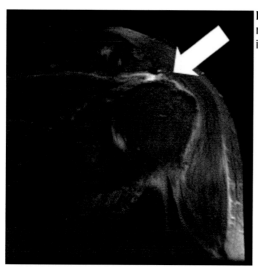

Figure 38-1. MRI showing full-thickness supraspinatus tear with moderate retraction. White arrow indicates retracted tear.

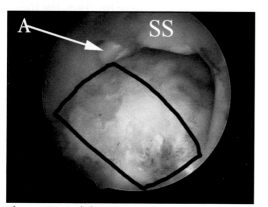 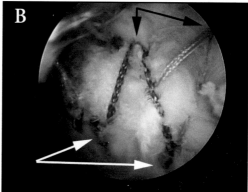

Figure 38-2. (A) Arthroscopic image of the patient in Figure 38-1 shows supraspinatus tear at surgery. "SS" Indicates torn edge of supraspinatus. Black box outlines native supraspinatus footprint. (B) Double-row suture-bridge repair of same tear. Black arrows show the medial row of suture anchors, passed in horizontal mattress configuration. Two lateral row anchors (white arrows) capture medial row sutures for compression against the footprint.

7. Warner JJP, Tetreault P, Lehtinen J, Zurakowski D. Arthroscopic versus mini-open rotator cuff repair: A cohort comparison study. *Arthroscopy*. 2005;21:328-332.
8. Galatz LM, Ball CM, Teefey SA, Middleton WD, Yamaguchi K. The outcome and repair integrity of completely arthroscopically repaired large and massive rotator cuff tears. *J Bone Joint Surg Am*. 2004;86:219-224.
9. Lee E, Bishop JY, Braman JP, Langford J, Gelber J, Flatow EL. Outcomes after arthroscopic rotator cuff repairs. *J Shoulder Elbow Surg*. 2007;16:1-5.

SECTION VIII

INSTABILITY QUESTIONS

39

How Do You Evaluate a Patient for a Posterior Dislocation After a Shoulder Trauma? If Dislocated, What Is Your Preferred Treatment?

R. Bryan Butler, MD
Anand Murthi, MD

Historically, most posterior dislocations have been associated with epileptic seizures, high-energy trauma, and, more infrequently now, electrocution or electroconvulsive treatment. Without history of trauma, posterior dislocation nearly always is associated with seizure, hypoglycemia, epilepsy, or alcohol withdrawal. The traumatic dislocation occurs when the arm is in a flexed, adducted, and internally rotated position. With seizures, the dislocation is instigated by sustained contracture of the internal rotators.

When ruling out posterior dislocation, the constant findings include an increased palpable prominence of the coracoid, a decreased palpable anterior prominence of the humeral head, an increased palpable posterior prominence below the acromion, marked limitation of abduction, and complete absence of external rotation. A fixed internal rotation deformity between 10 and 60 degrees is the rule.[1]

Similarly, 5 keys to conducting a physical examination that provides the diagnosis are as follows:

1. Examine the patient in the standing and sitting positions.

2. Ask the patient to flex both elbows to 90 degrees (with forearm directly anterior) so that you will see the fixed internal rotation deformity of the posterior dislocation.

3. When extending the arms, the patient with a posterior dislocation will be unable to turn the palm upward on the affected side because although the forearm is in complete supination, the shoulder is locked in internal rotation, thus preventing the palm from turning upward.

4. Observe the patient from above to note the absence of the anterior contour of the shoulder and the presence of posterior fullness in a posterior dislocation.

5. When the patient's arm is elevated, the angle of the scapula is felt to move immediately, indicating locking of the humeral head on the glenoid rim.[2]

Last, patients with shoulder trauma presenting from other physicians, such as after an emergency department visit, usually are positioned in a sling with the arm adducted and internally rotated (as most slings place the arm). Thus, the delayed presentation—or any presentation with a patient in a sling—can mask a locked posterior dislocation and should always be critically evaluated.

An adequate trauma radiograph series is necessary and will provide sufficient information. The series must include an axillary lateral view. If the patient cannot abduct his or her arm to achieve an adequate axillary view, a Velpeau lateral view can be substituted. If radiographs are inadequate or further assessment of the amount of humeral head involvement is needed, computed tomography (CT) is performed.

Once the diagnosis is established, appropriate treatment must be initiated. Dislocations that are acute (recognized within the first 2 to 3 weeks after injury) deserve a trial of closed reduction. If the dislocation is acute and the anterior humeral defect (known as the *reverse Hill-Sachs lesion*) is estimated to be less than 25% of the articular surface, we attempt closed reduction with the patient under anesthesia, with traction applied along the axis of the humerus (to disengage the defect), along with gentle external rotation and a push against the humeral head from posterior. Once reduced, the shoulder is examined for instability. If the defect is less than 25%, the shoulder usually remains stable and does not redislocate. We then place the arm in a "gunslinger" position, with the shoulder slightly extended, abducted approximately 15 degrees, and in neutral to slight external rotation (avoiding internal rotation). The position is maintained for 4 to 6 weeks before passive motion exercises are begun, with avoidance of flexion and internal rotation for 3 months.

If, however, the defect is larger and the shoulder is unstable after reduction, or if the shoulder is irreducible and the defect is estimated to be greater than 50%, we perform open reduction through a deltopectoral approach. During open reduction, it is important to release the posterior capsule. If reduction is achieved, the shoulder should be checked for stability. If the injury is acute and the defect is small (less than 25%) yet unstable after reduction, we disimpact the defect and re-enforce it with cancellous autograft or allograft chips. When making a cortical bone window through the greater tuberosity opposite the defect, we use a bone tamp or osteotome to impact the bone below the articular surface of the defect. Once we visualize the restored articular surface, the void of disimpacted bone below the subchondral bone is filled with bone graft and the cortical window is closed.

If disimpaction is prohibited because the injury is older and more sclerotic (ie, older than 2 to 3 weeks) yet the defect is smaller, we use the McLaughlin procedure[1] or the Neer modification of the McLaughlin procedure[3] (when an associated lesser tuberosity fracture is present) and transfer the subscapularis tendon (and/or the lesser tuberosity) into the anterior humeral head defect, essentially making the cavitary lesion "extracapsular" and unable to engage the glenoid rim. If the defect is larger but less than 40% to 50%, we use structural allograft or autograft secured with screws to fill the defect (Figure 39-1).

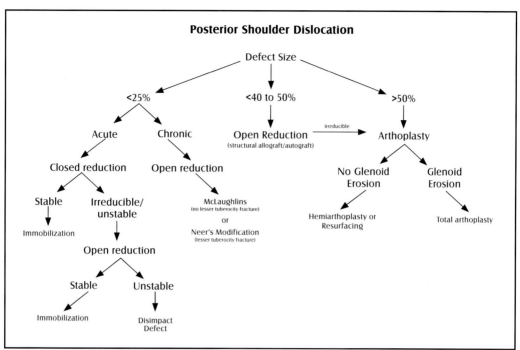

Figure 39-1. Algorithm of treatment options for posterior shoulder dislocations based on duration (acute, <2 to 3 weeks; chronic, >3 weeks) from injury to presentation and percent (%) of articular surface involvement of the humeral head defect.

Larger lesions (greater than 50%), regardless of chronicity, almost always are treated with arthroplasty, either hemi- or total. Only on rare occasions, we will consider preserving the head with structural bone graft when a younger person has great bone quality, no evidence of arthrosis, and a large defect present. Otherwise, the treatment of choice is hemiarthroplasty if no evidence of glenoid erosion is present or total arthroplasty if evidence of glenoid arthrosis is present (Figures 39-2 to 39-4). Resurfacing hemiarthroplasty also has been successful in our limited series.[4]

Posterior dislocations should be diagnosed acutely because they present with classic findings. Furthermore, the more chronic the dislocation is, the more limited your options will be as closed reduction becomes more difficult, the cavitary defect becomes larger and more sclerotic, and the capsule becomes tighter. Therefore, it is important to treat the defects as soon as possible, and if performed correctly, closed reduction will be appropriate. However, if closed reduction is attempted, plans for other possible procedures that include soft-tissue reconstruction, the use of allograft or autograft, and the use of a prosthetic replacement must be in place. It is important that the patient be aware of all the possibilities before you perform the planned intervention.

Figure 39-2. Anteroposterior view radiograph of a 51-year-old female patient after a fall, presenting 5 weeks after her injury; the image shows the typical "light-bulb" sign (caused by the internal rotation of the humerus) of a locked posterior dislocation.

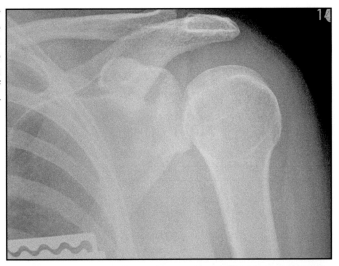

Figure 39-3. Axillary lateral view radiograph shows the posterior dislocation and the large, glenoid-engaging, humeral head defect (reverse Hill-Sachs lesion).

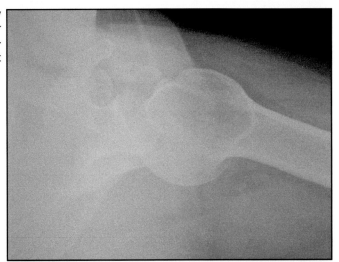

Figure 39-4. Postoperative radiograph of a hemiarthroplasty performed on the same patient who had a chronic posterior dislocation with a humeral head defect greater than 50% of the articular surface.

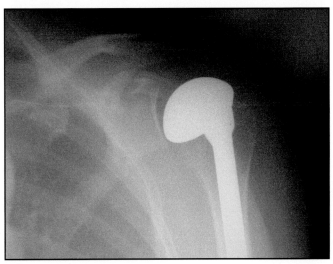

References

1. McLaughlin HL. Posterior dislocation of the shoulder. *J Bone Joint Surg Am.* 1952;34:584-590.
2. Rowe CR, Zarins B. Chronic unreduced dislocations of the shoulder. *J Bone Joint Surg Am.* 1982;64:494-505.
3. Hawkins RJ, Neer CS II, Pianta RM, Mendoza FX. Locked posterior dislocation of the shoulder. *J Bone Joint Surg Am.* 1987;69:9-18.
4. O'Brien M, Donaldson CT, Stein JA. Shoulder resurfacing arthroplasty in the young patient. Presented at the 74th Annual Meeting of the American Academy of Orthopaedic Surgeons. San Diego, CA, February 14-18, 2007.

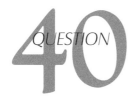

40

AT ARTHROSCOPY FOR ANTERIOR INSTABILITY, THERE IS AN "INVERTED-PEAR" GLENOID, OR 20% TO 25% LOSS OF THE ANTEROINFERIOR GLENOID. WHAT WOULD BE THE BEST RECONSTRUCTIVE OPTION WITH THIS INTRAOPERATIVE FINDING?

Matthew D. Williams, MD
T. Bradley Edwards, MD

Although we always try to know by history, physical examination, and imaging studies the osseous status of the glenohumeral joint in instability, there are times when we are surprised by the arthroscopic findings. We are always cognizant of the possibility of anteroinferior glenoid bone erosion or loss in these instability cases. The normal shape of the glenoid is that of a pear—wider inferiorly than superiorly. Recurrent instability with subluxation or frank dislocation over time causes wear of the antero-inferior glenoid. Once 20% to 25% of the rim has been eroded, the shape of the glenoid takes on the appearance of an inverted pear—wider superiorly than inferiorly. The alteration in glenoid form affects surgical outcomes following operative intervention for recurrent instability.

In our practice, patients with recurrent anterior instability are evaluated clinically and radiographically with a glenoid profile view of both shoulders as described by Bernageau and colleagues.[1] Bone loss appreciated radiographically is an indication for open stabilization using the Latarjet procedure.[2] Transfer of the coracoid bone block effectively restores glenohumeral stability without compromising external rotation. Should a bony lesion not be identified on preoperative imaging and we discover an inverted-pear glenoid arthroscopically, the arthroscopic procedure is abandoned and we perform a Latarjet procedure.

There are few contraindications to performing a Latarjet procedure: tears of the sub-scapularis and glenoid fractures involving greater than one-third of the articular surface. Large anterior glenoid rim fractures should be fixed primarily. Fractures that are not repairable require reconstruction; we use autologous iliac crest bone graft in this situation.

Arthroscopic and open glenohumeral stabilization procedures have been reported extensively in the literature and demonstrate roughly equivalent success rates in patients without bone loss as a contributing factor to their instability. However, arthroscopic stabilization of patients with bone loss has a reported failure (ie, episodes of recurrent instability) rate of 14% to 67%.[3,4] Burkhart and DeBeer[3] reported on 194 consecutive arthroscopic Bankart repairs. Patients without bone defects had a recurrence rate of 4% in contrast to 67% of those with glenoid bone loss. Mologne and colleagues[4] evaluated patients undergoing arthroscopic anterior stabilization with inverted-pear glenoids. The recurrence rate in this cohort of patients was 14%. Although the arthroscopic Bankart repair is the accepted gold standard treatment for anterior instability without associated bone loss, the presence of bone lesions decreases its efficacy as a treatment option.

Hovelius and colleagues[5] reported on over 100 patients treated with a coracoid transfer procedure for recurrent anterior instability. Seventy-two of these patients had a documented Bankart lesion. Over a 15-year follow-up, the recurrence rate was 3.4%. The patients able to return to sports in this report, including contact activities, was 86%.

Although the Latarjet is a nonanatomic procedure typically described as a "bone block," the coracoid fragment does not directly prevent subluxation. The coracoid bone block fills the glenoid defect and effectively increases the surface area of the glenoid. The second stabilizing effect is provided by the conjoined tendon, which provides an anteroinferior soft-tissue bumper when the shoulder is abducted and externally rotated. Suturing the capsule and inferior glenohumeral ligament to a stump of coracoacromial ligament transferred with the coracoid provides the third stabilizing mechanism, similar to that in a conventional Bankart procedure. Therefore, the Latarjet procedure provides a "triple block" to anterior glenohumeral instability (Figure 40-1).

The Latarjet is a technically demanding procedure and successful results depend on proper technique. Coracoid fracture is a devastating complication caused by overtightening of the lag screws. Nonunion of the coracoid to the glenoid results most often from soft-tissue interposition in the bony interface. Nonunion may be avoided by adequate exposure and retraction of the subscapularis during the procedure. Postoperative arthritis is associated with lateral overhang of the coracoid fragment over the glenoid rim. The coracoid must be placed flush with or medial to the glenoid rim and its final position checked at the time of surgery. External rotation loss and stiffness are often cited as drawbacks to performing this procedure. However, these complications are rare and unlikely with appropriate technique.

Rehabilitation following the Latarjet begins with 1 to 2 weeks in a simple sling. Active range of motion activities start the first day following surgery as tolerated by the patient. We clear patients to return to full activity, including contact sports, at 3 months postoperatively.

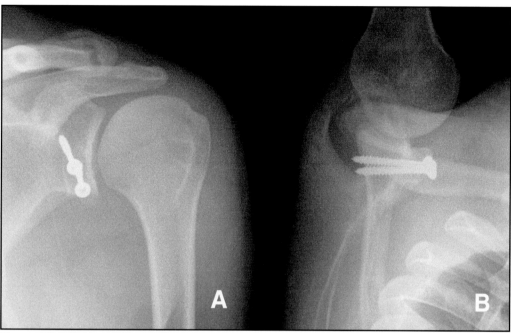

Figure 40-1. Postoperative radiographs of an 18-year-old athlete with recurrent anterior glenohumeral instability treated with a Latarjet coracoid transfer procedure. Anteroposterior view (A) and axillary view (B) showing proper fixation of the coracoid with two 4.5-mm malleolar screws and positioning medial to the glenoid rim.

References

1. Bernageau J, Patte D, Bebeyre J, Ferrane J. Intérêt du profil glénoidien dans les luxations récidivantes de l'épaule. *Rev Chir Orthop.* 1976;62(Suppl II):142-147.
2. Edwards TB, Walch G. The Latarjet procedure for recurrent anterior shoulder instability: rationale and technique. *Oper Tech Sports Med.* 2002;10:25-32.
3. Burkhart SS, DeBeer JF. Traumatic glenohumeral bone defects and their relationship to failure of arthroscopic Bankart repairs: significance of the inverted-pear glenoid and the humeral engaging Hill-Sachs lesion. *Arthroscopy.* 2000;16:677-694.
4. Mologne TS, Provencher MT, Menzel KA, Vachon TA, Dewing CB. Arthroscopic stabilization in patients with an inverted pear glenoid: results in patients with bone loss of the anterior glenoid. *Am J Sports Med.* Epub ahead of print, 2007.
5. Hovelius L, Sandstrom B, Sundgren K, Saebo M. One hundred eighteen Bristow-Latarjet repairs for recurrent anterior dislocation of the shoulder prospectively followed for fifteen years: study I—clinical results. *J Shoulder Elbow Surg.* 2004;13:509-516.

WHAT ARE THE TYPICAL FINDINGS IN A PATIENT WITH POSTERIOR INSTABILITY AND WHAT ARE THE INDICATIONS FOR OPEN VERSUS ARTHROSCOPIC POSTERIOR INSTABILITY REPAIR IN A HIGH SCHOOL OFFENSIVE LINEMAN?

A. Dushi Parameswaran, MD
Matthew T. Provencher, MD, LCDR, MC, USNR

The most frequent etiology of recurrent posterior instability is repetitive microtrauma. This is most often seen in sporting activities that involve repetitive loading of the glenohumeral joint while forward of the body. This includes football (blocking activities), volleyball, baseball, softball, rowing, and swimming, all of which position the shoulder in a flexed, adducted, internally rotated position, which places the posterior band of the inferior glenohumeral ligament (IGHL) on stretch.[1-5] We maintain an index of suspicion for posterior instability in young athletes with shoulder pain that is present during flexion/internal rotation activities, and reproduced in the clinic with certain physical examination maneuvers.

These activities repetitively injure the posteroinferior capsulolabral complex and contribute to a loss of glenoid-labral continuity,[6] injure the posterior labrum, and stretch the posterior IGHL.

We feel that the diagnosis of posterior instability is more difficult than making the diagnosis of anterior instability, because it is not as obvious and can masquerade as or coincide with other conditions of the shoulder. Often, patients may be referred with nonspecific complaints of shoulder pain, discomfort, weakness, and loss of athletic

Figure 41-1. Testing a patient with suspected posterior instability in the clinic. The patient is in the lateral decubitus position, with the scapula well stabilized by the examiners hip. The humerus is placed in a provocative position (flexion and internal rotation) and stress is applied to the posteroinferior capsulolabral complex to assess for reproduction of instability complaints.

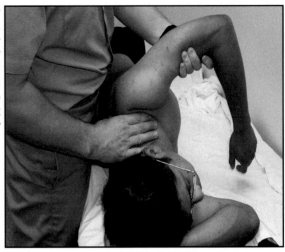

performance.[1-3] A comprehensive physical examination is one of the most important aspects in the evaluation of a patient with suspected posterior instability of the shoulder. Both shoulders should be examined, observing any obvious dislocation, asymmetry, abnormal motion, muscle atrophy, swelling, and scapular winging and maltracking. Scapulothoracic dyskinesis should be carefully evaluated. The asymptomatic shoulder may be examined first to gain patient confidence and relaxation. Provocative maneuvers allow the physician to determine the direction and degree of instability. The posterior apprehension or stress test may reproduce the specific shoulder symptoms; however, apprehension is not usually demonstrated by patients with posterior instability and should alert the physician that the shoulder may be subluxating anteriorly.[3] Other important posterior instability tests include the jerk test, the posterior stress test, the Kim test,[7] and the load and shift test, all of which stress the posteroinferior capsuloligamentous complex. We prefer to evaluate clinical instability in the lateral decubitus position on the examination table, stabilizing the posterior aspect of the capsule with the hip and maneuvering the humerus with both hands (Figure 41-1). The key finding is the reproduction of symptoms with the glenohumeral joint in a flexed and internally rotated position.

Radiographic and magnetic resonance imaging (MRI) studies usually demonstrate a posteroinferior labral tear, or, in the case of an MRI arthrogram, the finding of a patulous posteroinferior capsule (Figure 41-2). Regardless, any findings on MRI need to be confirmed with a clinical examination demonstrating symptomatic instability. We try to correlate the history, the physical examination findings, imaging findings, examination under anesthesia findings, and the arthroscopic findings into an operative treatment plan at the time of surgery. We expect the unexpected in this diagnostic category.

Operative stabilization should only be considered in patients with limited function of the involved shoulder secondary to pain and/or instability, who are psychologically stable and have failed an adequate trial of conservative therapy. Surgical treatment should only be offered for clear findings of instability (reproduction of symptoms with humeral translation) and not merely the finding of laxity (normal joint motion and translation without symptoms). In posterior instability, there may also be a "voluntary" component that is due more to positional control (flexed and internally rotated is able to subluxate

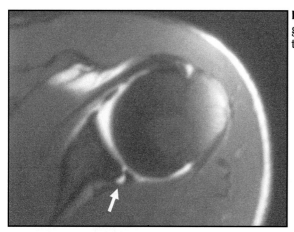

Figure 41-2. A magnetic resonance arthrogram demonstrating a posterior labral tear.

the shoulder) and does not necessarily portend a poor outcome as is the finding in multidirectional instability.

The results of open treatment of posterior instability have not fared very well, likely due to the large surgical dissection, and biomechanical properties of the posteroinferior capsule and labrum that are different from that of the anterior aspect of the shoulder.[3] Hawkins and colleagues[3] reported an overall recurrence rate of 50% utilizing 3 different open procedures.

The advantages of arthroscopic treatment include less operative dissection and the ability to address concomitant pathology and access the posterior capsulolabral complex. However, successful arthroscopic treatment is predicated on reproducing open surgical techniques with arthroscopic means. Due to these increased technical demands, there are several challenging areas to address when managing patients with posterior instability arthroscopically.

An arthroscopic capsular plication[8] is a surgical technique that imbricates and closes down the patulous pouch of the shoulder with a suture (absorbable or nonabsorbable), using the fixation point as an intact glenoid labrum. This is in contrast to a capsulolabral repair with anchors, which utilizes the glenoid anchor as the fixation point. The decision to perform an anchor repair versus a capsular plication is not well defined; however, it is generally felt that those with an intact labrum are amenable to capsular plication without anchors as long as the posteroinferior glenoid labrum is completely intact. The labrum has been shown to be a solid fixation point[9]; however, concerns of shear stress, small labral tear propagation, an unrecognized Kim lesion, and suture breakage may serve as indications for anchor fixation, which remains the strongest and most predictable repair construct (Figure 41-3).

We prefer a capsulolabral repair of the posteroinferior quadrant of the shoulder, generally from the 6 o'clock to the 10 o'clock position (for a right shoulder), utilizing 3 to 4 anchors spaced evenly about 5 to 7 mm apart. With the arthroscope in the anterosuperior portal, the repair is accomplished after establishing an accessory posterolateral portal (7 o'clock portal) to assist with anchor placement, suture management, and repair. A variety of repair devices are utilized from either the posterior or accessory posterior portal, and approximately 1 cm of capsule (depending upon magnitude of injury) is repaired to the labrum, which may be either intact, partially torn (Kim lesion), or fully torn (Figure

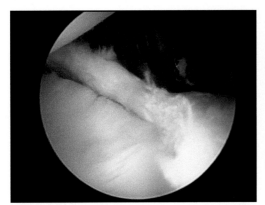 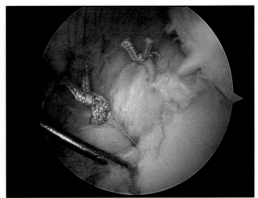

Figure 41-3. Arthroscopic view from the anterosuperior portal demonstrating a posterior labral tear, comprising the posteroinferior labrum (6 o'clock to approximately 2 o'clock).

Figure 41-4. Completed posterior labral repair. A total of 3 glenoid anchors were utilized with simple vertical capsulolabral repair sutures (each suture accomplishing about a 1 cm capsular plication repair).

41-4). We have found that the majority of patients with posterior instability have a completely torn labrum from approximately 6 to 10 o'clock.

The role of the rotator interval in posterior instability of the shoulder is frequently discussed and the decision to perform an arthroscopic rotator interval closure remains a challenge in patients with posterior instability. Recent biomechanical evidence[10] has suggested that arthroscopic rotator interval closure is not very beneficial in posterior shoulder instability. In addition, many surgeons have not closed the rotator interval in posterior instability[4] and have obtained satisfactory results, without the potential external rotation loss that has been described biomechanically.[10-11] There is no clear evidence that it adds to the stability of the shoulder; however, in selected cases of excessive laxity[19,20] after adequate capsulolabral repair, it may be a useful adjunct.

An abduction sling is utilized for 5 to 6 weeks, starting first with passive Codman exercises, progressing to passive range of motion (ROM) in the scapular plane, and then active assisted ROM by 4 to 6 weeks. Terminal stretching is then completed at 6 to 8 weeks, followed by a strengthening program emphasizing the scapular stabilizers and internal rotators. Sports participation is allowed at around 4 to 6 months, depending upon the level of contact.

Although the results of arthroscopic treatment of posterior shoulder instability continue to improve,[1-3] the overall efficacy has not been as encouraging as those treated for unidirectional anterior instability. This is due to patient selection, the inherent biomechanical differences of the posteroinferior capsulolabral complex, and unrecognized pathology. Overall, recent results of arthroscopic treatment are encouraging, although longer-term studies are needed to truly assess the efficacy of these procedures.

References

1. Bottoni CR, Franks BR, Moore JH, DeBerardino TM, Taylor DC, Arciero RA. Operative stabilization of posterior shoulder instability. *Am J Sports Med.* 2005;33:996-1002.
2. Bradley JP, Baker CL 3rd, Kline AJ, Armfield DR, Chhabra A. Arthroscopic capsulolabral reconstruction for posterior instability of the shoulder: a prospective study of 100 shoulders. *Am J Sports Med.* 2006;34:1061-1071.
3. Hawkins R, Koppert G, Johnston G. Recurrent posterior instability (subluxation) of the shoulder. *J Bone Joint Surg Am.* 1984;66A:169-174.
4. Provencher MT, Bell SJ, Menzel KA, Mologne TS. Arthroscopic Treatment of Posterior Shoulder Instability. Results in 33 Patients. *Am J Sports Med.* 2005;33(10):1463-71.
5. Provencher MT, King S, Solomon D, Bell SJ, Mologne TS. Recurrent posterior shoulder instability: Diagnosis and management. *Oper Tech Sports Med.* 2005;13(4):196-205.
6. Kim S, Noh K, Park J, Ryu B, Oh I. Loss of chondrolabral containment of the glenohumeral joint in atraumatic posteroinferior multidirectional instability. *J Bone Joint Surg Am.* 2005;87:92-98.
7. Kim S, Park J, Jeong W, Shin S. The Kim test: A novel test for posteroinferior labral lesion of the shoulder—a comparison to the jerk test. *Am J Sports Med.* 2005;33:1188-1192.
8. Hewitt M, Getelman MH, Snyder SJ. Arthroscopic management of multidirectional instability: pancapsular plication. *Orthop Clin North Am.* 2003;34:549-557.
9. Provencher MT, Verma N, Obopilwe E, Rincon LM, Tracy J, Romeo AA, Mazzocca A. A biomechanical analysis of capsular plication versus anchor repair of the shoulder: can the labrum be used as a suture anchor? *Arthroscopy.* 2008;24(2):210-216.
10. Provencher MT, Mologne TS, Michio H, Zhao K, Tasto JP, An KN. Arthroscopic versus open rotator interval closure: biomechanical evaluation of stability and motion. *Arthroscopy.* 2007;23(6):583-592.
11. Antoniou J, Duckworth DT, Harryman DT 2nd. Capsulolabral augmentation for the management of posteroinferior instability of the shoulder. *J Bone Joint Surg Am.* 2000;82A:1220-1230.

HOW DO YOU MANAGE A HIGH SCHOOL QUARTERBACK WHO DISLOCATES HIS THROWING SHOULDER (FIRST TIME DISLOCATION) IN THE FIRST GAME OF THE SEASON? AND HOW DO YOU MANAGE A COLLEGE DIVISION 1 QUARTERBACK WHO DISLOCATES HIS SHOULDER IN THE FIRST GAME OF THE SEASON?

John-Erik Bell, MD
Christopher S. Ahmad, MD

These clinical scenarios can be broken down into 3 separate considerations: (1) indications for surgery versus nonoperative treatment, (2) timing of surgical intervention, and (3) arthroscopic versus open treatment stabilization in a contact athlete. We would obtain standard x-ray views and magnetic resonance imaging (MRI) scans to document the pathology. Assuming the predicted pathology is an anterior inferior labral tear, there remain 4 choices for management of this clinical scenario, regardless of the level of athletic competition—high school amateur, Division 1 collegiate, or professional.[1] The first is to complete the season and postpone surgery until the off-season. The second is to continue competing until a recurrence occurs, and then proceed to surgery. The third is to sacrifice the current season and undergo primary surgical reconstruction. The fourth choice is to complete the season and forgo surgical treatment altogether in favor of off-season rehabilitation.

Since the classic paper in which Arciero and colleagues initially demonstrated in convincing fashion that patient age is the most significant prognostic factor in predicting recurrence, many additional studies have found identical results.[2] Furthermore, several prospective randomized studies have compared directly immediate surgical reconstruction with nonoperative treatment in young athletes and found dramatically improved results in the group undergoing surgery.[3-5] These studies certainly support surgical reconstruction for the high-level athlete after a single anterior dislocation, given the extremely high risk of recurrence and the potential loss of another subsequent season with nonoperative treatment.

Most competitive athletes, whether high school or college, do not want to sacrifice an entire season, as would be necessary if surgery was undertaken immediately following a dislocation in the first game of the season due to the lengthy postoperative rehabilitation protocol, which places restrictions on return to sport. Buss and colleagues reported on their experience with treating in-season athletes with anterior shoulder instability nonoperatively.[6] It was found that 90% were able to return for either part or all of their seasons, at the same or equivalent playing position at subjectively the same level of play, with an average of 1.4 recurrent instability episodes per athlete per season. One of the disadvantages cited by proponents of immediate operative intervention despite loss of the current season is that recurrent instability episodes create additional glenohumeral joint damage and that this can be prevented by earlier surgery. To our knowledge, improved outcomes as a result of avoiding additional dislocations have never been demonstrated.

Our approach to both quarterbacks presented in this question would be similar regarding indications and timing of surgery. For the Division 1 collegiate quarterback, we would present to the athlete these options. It is our experience that the majority of high-performance athletes would choose to complete their season if possible. We do not immobilize the shoulder for more than a couple of days while the acute pain subsides. Our rehabilitation protocol for athletes wishing to return in the same season as their dislocation includes maintenance of range of motion (ROM), strengthening of the rotator cuff and scapular stabilizers, and return to competition when the injured extremity has symmetrical strength and ROM, allowing unrestricted play. We typically would utilize a shoulder neoprene brace for a quarterback in this scenario, which allows abduction and external rotation required for overhead throwing but may enhance protective shoulder proprioception.

The outcome will either be successful completion of the season or demonstration of recurrent instability that precludes continued play. In either of these situations, we would recommend surgical reconstruction of the high-level athlete at the completion of the season to minimize the potential loss of the following season due to recurrent instability, the chance of which is up to 94% in a competitive male contact athlete of age 21.[7] For the high school athlete, we would also consider the option of continued nonoperative care in the surgery-averse patient who on examination does not demonstrate a positive apprehension-relocation maneuver, but would be certain that the patient understood the high probability of recurrent dislocation in the following season in the under 20 age group without surgical reconstruction.

The second controversy inherent in this question is whether this collision sport athlete should be reconstructed using an open or arthroscopic technique. Traditional thinking was that open reconstructive procedures were more durable and more appropriate for

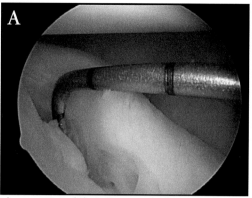 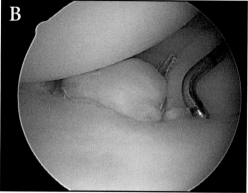

Figure 42-1. (A) Arthroscopic image of anterior inferior labral detachment. (B) Arthroscopic image of anterior inferior labrum fixed with suture anchor and nonabsorbable suture.

contact athletes, possibly because of increased scar formation and more secure fixation. However, recent reports indicate that arthroscopic treatment is also effective in contact athletes.[8] We prefer to treat contact athletes arthroscopically, provided that there is no significant glenoid bone deficiency, no engaging Hill-Sachs lesion on the humerus, and no evidence of a humeral avulsion of glenohumeral ligament (HAGL) lesion. For overhead athletes such as the quarterbacks in this question, we would prefer arthroscopic treatment to minimize loss of external rotation, which can significantly affect throwing velocity. We would then restrict the athlete from contact sports for 6 months postoperatively, but would fully expect recovery in time for the following season (Figure 42-1).

References

1. Burris MW, Johnson DL, Mair SD. Management of in-season anterior shoulder dislocation in the amateur athlete. *Orthopedics.* 2007;30:362-364.
2. Arciero RA, Wheeler JH, Ryan JB, McBride JT. Arthroscopic Bankart repair versus nonoperative treatment for acute, initial anterior shoulder dislocations. *Am J Sports Med.* 1994;22:589-594.
3. Jakobsen BW, Johannsen HV, Suder P, Sojbjerg JO. Primary repair versus conservative treatment of first-time traumatic anterior dislocation of the shoulder: a randomized study with 10-year follow-up. *Arthroscopy.* 2007; 23:118-123.
4. Kirkley A, Werstine R, Ratjek A, Griffin S. Prospective randomized clinical trial comparing the effectiveness of immediate arthroscopic stabilization versus immobilization and rehabilitation in first traumatic anterior dislocations of the shoulder: long-term evaluation. *Arthroscopy.* 2005;21:55-63.
5. Bottoni CR, Wilckens JH, DeBerardino TM, et al. A prospective, randomized evaluation of arthroscopic stabilization versus nonoperative treatment in patients with acute, traumatic, first-time shoulder dislocations. *Am J Sports Med.* 2002;30:576-580.
6. Buss DD, Lynch GP, Meyer CP, Huber SM, Freehill MQ. Nonoperative management for in-season athletes with anterior shoulder instability. *Am J Sports Med.* 2004;32:1430-1433.
7. Larrain MV, Botto GJ, Montenegro HJ, Mauas DM. Arthroscopic repair of acute traumatic anterior shoulder dislocation in young athletes. *Arthroscopy.* 2001;17:373-377.
8. Mazzocca AD, Brown FM Jr., Carreira DS, Hayden J, Romeo AA. Arthroscopic anterior shoulder stabilization of collision and contact athletes. *Am J Sports Med.* 2005;33:52-60.

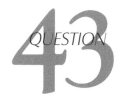

WHAT ARE THE PREFERRED MANAGEMENT OPTIONS AND WORK-UP FOR AN INDIVIDUAL WHO PRESENTS 1 YEAR AFTER A FAILED ARTHROSCOPIC INSTABILITY REPAIR?

Rodney J. Stanley, MD
T. Bradley Edwards, MD

Although arthroscopic treatment of anterior instability can be highly successful in properly selected patients, failures still occur. Reasons for failure include technical errors during the primary surgery, bone defects, hyperlaxity, and patient noncompliance.[1,2]

When we have a patient with recurrent instability after prior surgery, we take a stepwise approach. The patient evaluation should include history (did he or she frankly redislocate or only sublux?), physical examination, and plain radiographs. Imaging studies with plain radiographs and more advanced imaging studies such as computed tomography (CT) and magnetic resonance imaging (MRI) are necessary. Obtaining the operative note of previous surgery is very important. Important factors obtained from the history include inciting event, symptoms, previous surgical procedure, and operative findings. Instability that recurs after a discrete traumatic injury may be handled differently than instability that develops gradually with minimal or no trauma. In the traumatic group, instability may result from a new lesion, whereas a gradual recurrence may indicate improper patient selection or technical errors from the previous surgery. Many patients will have symptoms of continual instability, most obvious in those with dislocations requiring reduction. However, in some cases, pain will supersede any sensations of instability.

It is often helpful to review past operative reports. This gives information about the procedure performed plus any pathologic lesions that were identified and addressed at the time of surgery. For example, glenoid rim defects, large Hill-Sachs lesions, and failure to correct anteroinferior capsular laxity or rotator interval laxity are risk factors for recurrence of shoulder instability after arthroscopic Bankart repair.[1-3] This information helps us chose between open or arthroscopic revision surgeries.

Figure 43-1. Anteroinferior fracture of the glenoid rim shown on a glenoid profile radiograph.

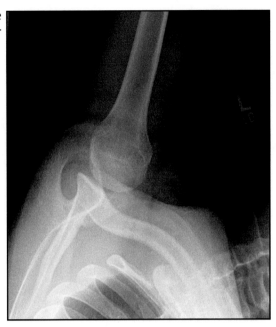

Physical examination is important in differentiating causes of recurrent instability. Positive anterior apprehension and relocation test results indicate clinical failure. Concomitant posterior or multidirectional instability should be ruled out. Anterior shoulder hyperlaxity is demonstrated by >90 degrees of external rotation with the arms at the side. This indicates a congenitally weak capsule, which is a risk factor for recurrence.[1] Scapular mechanics should be assessed and dyskinesia corrected before considering surgery.

Plain radiographs are useful in finding bone deficiencies associated with recurrent instability (Figure 43-1) and to assess placement and migration of metallic anchors. CT scans are a valuable adjunct for quantifying large glenoid rim defects or Hill-Sachs lesions. MRI, particularly with intra-articular contrast, can identify recurrent Bankart lesions, superior labral tears, medially healed Bankart lesions, capsular avulsions, capsular redundancy, and rotator cuff tears.

Examination under anesthesia (EUA) and intraoperative findings are used to verify the diagnosis at the time of repeat surgery. EUA will rule out posterior or multidirectional instability and demonstrate any anterior hyperlaxity. Diagnostic arthroscopy may be performed to evaluate glenoid bone stock, presence of superior labral tears, medially healed Bankart lesions, humeral avulsion of the glenohumeral ligament, and rotator cuff pathology.

Do not neglect the fact that the original rehabilitation may have been suboptimal. Rehabilitation should be maximized before considering revision surgery. This should include correction of soft-tissue contracture, rotator cuff weakness, and periscapular dysfunction. With recurrent anterior instability, the most common revision surgery options include repeat arthroscopic reconstruction, open Bankart repair, and Latarjet-Bristow procedures. Less commonly performed procedures include bone grafts for large Hill-Sachs defects, and allograft or autograft capsular reconstruction for significant soft-tissue deficiencies as seen following failed thermal capsulorraphy. The optimal procedure is

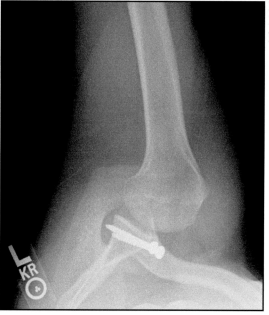

Figure 43-2. Glenoid profile radiograph after Latarjet procedure shows increased anterior posterior diameter of the glenoid fossa.

determined based on patient expectation, activity level, surgeon experience, and pathologic lesions leading to failure of the previous surgery.

Arthroscopic revision Bankart repair can be considered in patients without bone defects or hyperlaxity. We primarily reserve this option for patients who present as a result of technical errors at the initial surgery. A prospective series of 23 patients with failed Bankart repair were treated with arthroscopic revision and followed for a minimum of 24 months.[3] The revision surgery consisted of repair of the anterior labrum with suture anchors, capsular plication, and proximal shift of the inferior capsule. Rotator interval closure was added if the patient had a grade I or II sulcus sign preoperatively or significant capsular laxity after the Bankart repair. In 5 patients, failure of the primary surgery was believed to result from nonanatomic repair, with labral tissue fixed proximal or medial to the glenoid margin. Eighteen patients achieved a return to more than 90% of their preinjury activity level. Five patients had recurrent instability after revision with 1 dislocation, 2 subluxations, and 2 positive anterior apprehension signs. In properly selected patients, revision arthroscopic Bankart repair can provide satisfactory results.

Many surgeons prefer open revision procedures for treating failed instability repair, especially in cases of hyperlaxity or bone defects where arthroscopic repair is contraindicated.[1] A series of 30 patients with failed arthroscopic Bankart repairs were treated with revision open Bankart repair.[2] In 87% of patients, the failure of initial arthroscopic surgery was felt to result from improper anchor placement. Following revision, there were no recurrences of instability and 87% of patients returned to previous activity level.

Our preferred method of treatment for recurrent anterior instability with significant glenoid bone defects or hyperlaxity is with the Latarjet procedure (Figure 43-2). Advantages of this procedure include a very low recurrence rate with minimal, if any, loss of external rotation.[4] Earlier and more aggressive activity is allowed than with soft-tissue procedures, with return to full athletic activities at 3 months postoperative. The Latarjet procedure provides a "triple blocking" effect with the coracoid bone block, the conjoined tendon sling, and a capsulolabral reconstruction by repairing the capsule to the stump of the coracoacromial ligament. The Latarjet procedure was performed on 9 patients with failure of arthroscopic Bankart repair and provided a stable shoulder in all 9.[1]

References

1. Boileau P, Villalba M, Hery JY, Balg F, Ahrens P, Neyton L. Risk factors for recurrence of shoulder instability after arthroscopic Bankart repair. *J Bone Joint Surg Am*. 2006;88:1755-1763.
2. Sisto DJ. Revision of failed arthroscopic Bankart repairs. *Am J Sports Med*. 2007;35:537-541.
3. Kim SH, Ha KI, Kim YM. Arthroscopic revision Bankart repair: a prospective outcome study. *Arthroscopy*. 2002;18:469-482.
4. Edwards TB, Walch G. The Latarjet procedure for recurrent anterior shoulder instability: rationale and technique. *Oper Tech Sports Med*. 2002;10:25-32.

What Is the Optimal Placement of Suture Anchors in an Arthroscopic Anterior Instability Repair and How Much Capsular Tissue Should Be Tensioned in the Capsulolabral Repair?

Ed Glenn, MD

The optimal placement of suture anchors in arthroscopic anterior instability repair begins with proper portal placement. I prefer to perform instability repairs in the lateral decubitus position because of the ability to distract the humeral head from the glenoid, which greatly improves visualization. Two anterior arthroscopic portals are used for the repair: a high anterior portal placed at the level of the biceps tendon, and a low anterior (mid-glenoid) portal placed just superior to the superior border of the subscapularis tendon. The portals need to be placed slightly more lateral than traditional anterior portals in order to properly place the anchors at the glenoid rim. If the portals are created too medial, the angle of approach for anchor placement is too "flat," and the glenoid articular surface can be compromised when the pilot hole is drilled. I create the portals using spinal needle localization. With the low anterior (mid-glenoid) portal, I make sure that I can move the spinal needle easily to the anteroinferior glenoid rim before the portal is created.

I place a 6.25-mm clear cannula in the high anterior portal and an 8.25-mm cannula in the low anterior (mid-glenoid) portal. After complete liberation of the anterior glenoid labrum from the glenoid neck (as indicated by the visualization of the subscapularis muscle fibers medial to the labral tissue) to the 6 o'clock position inferiorly and a gentle debridement of soft tissue from the anterior glenoid neck, the anchors are ready to be placed.

The first anchor is placed as low as possible approximately 2 mm onto the anterior glenoid face,[1] about the 5:30 o'clock position on a right shoulder (6:30 o'clock position on a left shoulder). Do not place the anchor on the anterior glenoid neck. This position is too medial and will not allow you to properly reestablish the "bumper" effect of the anterior labrum. The anchor should be placed at a 45-degree angle to the articular surface of the glenoid. This won't be possible if the low anterior (mid-glenoid) portal is placed too medially. Once the anchor is placed, a single limb of suture is pulled through the high anterior portal. A suture shuttling device is then placed through the low anterior (mid-glenoid) portal to capture the anterior capsule and the anterior labrum. I capture the anterior capsule about 1 cm inferior and 1 cm lateral to the anchor. I then pull the captured capsule superiorly and medially and capture the anterior labrum at the level of the anchor. The suture in the suture shuttling device is then brought out the high anterior portal and tied to the suture limb from the suture anchor. The suture is then shuttled retrograde through the labrum and capsular tissue and pulled out the low anterior (mid-glenoid) portal.

The 2 suture limbs from the suture anchor are then tied together. The suture limb that was passed through the labrum and capsule should be the post strand in order to keep the knot off of the glenoid articular surface. By capturing the anterior capsular tissue inferior and lateral to the suture anchor, a superior and medial shift of the joint capsule is afforded in addition to the labral repair. This effectively reduces the anterior capsular volume to minimize the risk of recurrent shoulder dislocation. Depending on the size of the anterior labral tear, 1 or 2 additional anchors are placed in a similar fashion at the 4:30 and 3 o'clock positions. The anterior capsular tissue and labrum are captured in a similar fashion, and the sutures sequentially tied from inferior to superior.

Reference

1. Mazzocca AD, Brown FM Jr, Carreira DS, Hayden J, Romeo AA. Arthroscopic anterior shoulder stabilization of collision and contact athletes. *Am J Sports Med.* 2005;33:52-60.

How Do You Manage an Axillary Nerve Palsy After a Shoulder Dislocation?

Michael Freehill, MD

Management of an axillary nerve palsy after a shoulder dislocation brings both good news and challenging news. The good news is that the majority of these patients who sustain the axillary nerve injury following dislocation will get better with conservative management. The challenging news is those who do not get better may require surgical intervention. The key to management is identification of the injury. Anatomically speaking, we know that the axillary nerve is the terminal branch of the posterior cord and typically receives innervation from the 5th and 6th cervical nerve roots. In the case of dislocation, the nerve is at greater risk in the area where it runs obliquely across the inferior and lateral border of the subscapularis, crossing within 3 to 5 mm from its musculotendinous junction.[1]

The nerve then enters the quadrilateral space along the posterior aspect of the shoulder accompanied by the posterior humeral circumflex artery. It is in this region where the nerve is most likely injured in the case of anterior inferior glenohumeral dislocations. In cases of acute dislocation, it may be difficult to ascertain the integrity of the axillary nerve due to the patient's acute pain. However, many patients will describe a loss of sensation or numbness along the anterolateral deltoid when closely compared to the contralateral uninjured arm. Reexamination within 1 to 2 weeks of the acute injury will allow for a more thorough evaluation of the manual muscle testing grade of the deltoid, including the posterior, lateral, and anterior heads.

Once an axillary nerve injury has been identified, management should include an electromyography (EMG) nerve conduction study within the first 2 to 4 weeks following the clinical diagnosis. Examination of the entire upper extremity should be included to rule out the possibility of a subacute brachial plexus injury in which the primary finding could be the axillary nerve palsy. The patient should be followed conservatively for an additional 3 to 4 months, beginning with active assisted range of motion exercises and isometric strengthening as tolerated. A repeat EMG study should be obtained within 3 to 4 months after the initial injury to determine whether or not there is any evidence of neurological recovery. The expectation for nonoperative management is generally a complete functional recovery. Studies have shown that the rate of injury to the axillary nerve can vary between 10% and 50% with fractures and/or dislocation injuries to the shoulder girdle. Several early studies have demonstrated that the recovery can take 1 to 2 years and upwards of 90% of the patients will have a full recovery.[2]

If there is no evidence of any clinical recovery or improvement on EMG nerve conduction studies, surgical intervention can be considered between 3 and 6 months following the injury.[3-5] Studies have shown that intervention within this time period appears to yield a greater functional improvement when nerve grafting or neurolysis is performed. Cases of traumatic injury in which traction has been applied to the extremity a neuroma in continuity can occur over several centimeters. Treatment frequently involves a resection of the neuroma with sural nerve grafting. There may be additional scar tissue in the axillary recess that can cause entrapment of the axillary nerve in the zone of injury. These patients are likely to respond to neurolysis through the affected region. Studies presented on nerve grafting revealed 67% to 95% of patients have achieved grade 4 or 5 strength postoperatively. The common theme in these studies was early intervention within the first 6 to 12 months following the injury. Patients who underwent surgery greater than 1 year after injury did not have the degree of excellent functional recoveries as those treated earlier following their course of injury.

A magnetic resonance imaging (MRI) scan should be considered in patients over the age of 40 who have an acute shoulder dislocation. Frequently, rotator cuff injuries can occur in the face of dislocation and can be masked by the presence of an axillary nerve injury in which forward elevation and abduction can be limited in both cases. Generally, in younger patients who have acute rotator cuff tears, attention to the rotator cuff should be considered while awaiting recovery of the axillary nerve palsy. Arthroscopic approaches are less likely to cause any further damage to the deltoid. If an open procedure is performed, great care must be taken to avoid any further injury to the deltoid. This can include excessive traction if performing a mini-open approach or a potential complication of the deltoid split in a traditional open approach. As such, a traction suture should be placed at the distal apex of the deltoid split to avoid any potential injury to the recovering axillary nerve.

Overall, nonoperative management of the axillary nerve palsy is the mainstay of treatment following a shoulder dislocation. A great majority of these patients will recover with conservative management. Operative management in the form of neurolysis or nerve grafting has proved to be promising with reported functional recoveries. Overall, I would recommend an EMG study/nerve conduction study be performed 2 to 4 weeks following their injury, with a subsequent reexamination 3 to 4 months following the original injury to determine the extent of neurologic recovery. When discernable recovery is seen at 3 to 4 months, continued observation can be considered for an additional 3 to 4 months with a repeat EMG once again performed at that time. If no functional improvement is noted clinically or electric-diagnostically, then neurolysis and possible nerve grafting should be considered as a viable treatment option.

References

1. Steinmann S, Moran E. Axillary nerve injury: diagnosis and treatment. *J Am Acad Orthop Surg.* 2001;9:328-335.
2. Blom S, Dahlback LO. Nerve injuries in dislocations of the shoulder joint and fractures of the neck of the humerus: a clinical and electromyographical study. *Acta Chir Scand.* 1970;136:461-466.
3. Perkins G, Watson Jones R. Fractures in the region of the shoulder joint. *Proc R Soc Med.* 1936;29:1055-1072.
4. Alnot JY, Valenti P. Surgical repair of the axillary nerve: apropos of 37 cases (in French). *Int Orthop.* 1991;15:7-11.
5. Coene LN, Narakas AO. Operative management of lesions of the axillary nerve, isolated or combined with other nerve lesions. *Clin Neurol Neurosurg.* 1992;94(suppl):S64-S66.

46

WHEN IS ARTHROSCOPIC CLOSURE OF THE ROTATOR INTERVAL INDICATED IN THE SETTING OF SHOULDER INSTABILITY— ANTERIOR, POSTERIOR, MULTIDIRECTIONAL?

Matthew T. Provencher, MD, LCDR, MC, USNR

The role of the rotator interval in shoulder instability remains controversial. Defined as the tissue between the supraspinatus (SS) and subscapularis (SSc) tendons, the rotator interval contains several anatomic structures, including the coracohumeral ligament (CHL), the superior glenohumeral ligament (SGHL), and the joint capsule (Figure 46-1). Many studies have assessed the influence of the rotator interval and have concluded that the rotator interval is important in maintaining both inferior and posterior stability of the glenohumeral joint.[1-5]

With the advancements in the arthroscopic treatment of shoulder instability, several authors have advocated the addition of a rotator interval closure to the standard arthroscopic anteroinferior capsulolabral repair to improve stabilization of the glenohumeral joint. Several authors advocate closure of the rotator interval as an adjunct to multidirectional and posterior instability repair. However, much of the thought regarding rotator interval closure is based on an elegant study performed by Harryman and colleagues in 1992, where an open imbrication of the rotator interval was performed, and they demonstrated improved posterior and inferior stability after rotator interval repair. However, an arthroscopic closure of the rotator interval is generally a cephalad shift of the middle glenohumeral ligament (MGHL) to the SGHL or capsule just anterior to the SS tendon, although variations of the rotator interval closure to the SS and/or the SSc tendons have been described. It should be kept in mind that the arthroscopic closure is different from the open closure as defined by Harryman and colleagues, and should not be applied to what is performed arthroscopically.[1,2]

Figure 46-1. (A and B) Rotator interval contents: the coracohumeral ligament, long head biceps, superior glenohumeral ligament, and long head of the biceps tendon. (Reprinted with permission from Matthew T. Provencher, MD.)

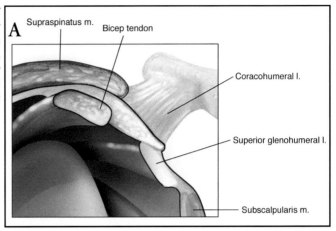

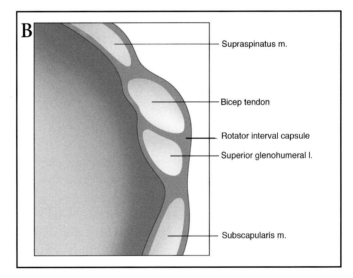

The effects of arthroscopic rotator interval closure have been assessed and reported in several studies,[1-5] which have demonstrated no improvement in posterior and inferior stability of the glenohumeral joint. However, there is a consistent improvement in anterior stability of the glenohumeral joint, probably due to a cephalad shift of the MGHL to either the SGHL or SS tendon, depending upon closure method.

Based on our work[1,2] and others[3] who have documented no benefit in posterior and inferior stability of the shoulder joint, we do not advocate the routine closure of the rotator interval. It should be kept in mind that the closure of the rotator interval is probably not without consequence, with a consistent decrease in external rotation at the side after interval repair, even when repaired with the arm in 30 degrees external rotation. However, rotator interval repair may serve as an adjunct to certain cases of anterior instability repair, such as in a revision situation, with lax or poor anterior tissue, and other conditions where a potential loss of external rotation can be tolerated (Figure 46-2).

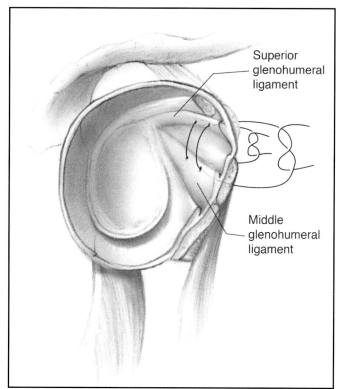

Superior
glenohumeral
ligament

Middle
glenohumeral
ligament

Figure 46-2. Typical rotator interval repair with two sutures 1 cm apart (medial to lateral separation), closing the middle and superior glenohumeral ligaments. (Reprinted with permission from Matthew T. Provencher, MD, LCDR, MC, USNR.)

References

1. Provencher MT, Mologne TS, Hongo M, Zhao K, Tasto JP, An KN. Arthroscopic versus open rotator interval closure: biomechanical evaluation of stability and motion. *Arthroscopy.* 2007;23:583-592.
2. Mologne TS, Zhao K, Hongo M, Romeo AA, An KN, Provencher MT. The addition of rotator interval closure after arthroscopic repair of either anterior or posterior shoulder instability: impact of glenohumeral translation and range of motion. Am J Sports Med. 2008; in press.
3. Plausinis D, Bravman JT, Heywood C, et al. Arthroscopic rotator interval closure: effect of sutures on glenohumeral motion and anterior-posterior translation. *Am J Sports Med.* 2006;34:1656-1661.
4. Wolf R, Zheng N, Iero J, Weichel D. The effects of thermal capsulorrhaphy and rotator interval closure on multidirectional laxity in the glenohumeral joint: a cadaveric biomechanical study. *Arthroscopy.* 2004;20:1044-1049.
5. Yamamoto N, Itoi E, Tuoheti Y, Seki N, Abe H, Minagawa H, Shimada Y, Okada K. Effect of rotator interval closure on glenohumeral stability and motion: a cadaveric study. *J Shoulder Elbow Surg.* 2006;15(6):750-758.

SECTION IX

ACROMIOCLAVICULAR QUESTIONS

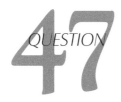

QUESTION

47

How Do You Manage an Acute Grade III Acromioclavicular Separation and When Do You Allow Return to Work and/or Sport? What Are the Indications for Surgical Reconstruction of AC Separation?

Clifford G. Rios, MD
Robert A. Arciero, MD
Anthony A. Romeo, MD
Augustus D. Mazzocca, MD

Traditionally, the management of type I and type II acromioclavicular (AC) joint separations has been supportive, with rest and anti-inflammatory medication, and return to motion and activity as symptoms reside. This treatment generally provides good results, although reports exist that describe poor outcomes with conservative treatment, which are improved following operative intervention. The more severe injuries, namely type IV or greater, are typically repaired or reconstructed with one of several techniques. Management of the patient with a type III AC separation is more controversial. This injury is characterized by complete disruption of both the AC and coracoclavicular (CC) ligaments, without much disruption of the deltoid or trapezial fascia. Clinically, the patient presents with a "high-riding" clavicle, which appears elevated due to relative depression of the acromion and upper extremity.

There are several factors that you must consider before determining if a patient with a type III AC separation should be managed operatively or nonoperatively. These include hand dominance, occupational or sporting requirements, presence of scapulothoracic

Figure 47-1. We make an incision 3.5 cm from the AC joint starting at the posterior clavicle and head in a curvilinear fashion towards the coracoid along Langer's lines. We often angle the incision to allow full visualization of the AC joint laterally and coracoid process medially. (Reprinted with permission from Arthrex, Inc, Naples, FL.)

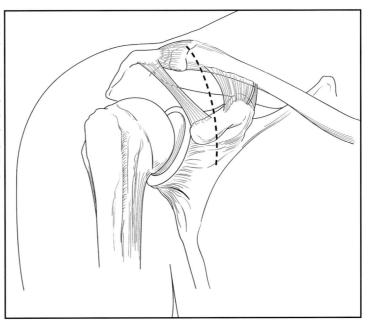

dysfunction, and the risk for reinjury. Unfortunately, the literature presents significant controversy regarding the need for anatomic reduction of the AC joint in a type III separation. Success rates in this population range from 87% to 96% in both operative and nonoperative treatment. Phillips and colleagues completed a meta-analysis of 1172 patients with type III injuries and identified 88% and 87% satisfactory outcomes in patients treated operatively and nonoperatively, respectively.[1] Studies of elite throwing athletes suggest that anatomic reduction of the AC joint is not necessary. Most surgeons will treat contact athletes nonoperatively due to the high risk of reinjury. Finally, when comparing operative and nonoperative intervention, it has been shown that there is no difference in strength with either treatment regimen 2 years postinjury. Thus, it is difficult to predict which patients will benefit from surgical intervention in this setting.

The authors have not treated any type III injuries with acute repair or reconstruction. Based on the available literature, we do not believe there is sufficient evidence to support surgical treatment of the acute type III AC separation.[2] We treat patients with an acute type III AC separation nonoperatively for 3 to 6 months. There is a subset of patients, however, who will have persistent pain and dysfunction that prevents return to work or sport. We offer surgical reconstruction to patients who have persistent symptoms despite a 3- to 6-month trial of rest and rehabilitation. We will operate on patients in the acute setting who have complete injuries (type IV or greater) due to the significant morbidity attributable to the dislocated joint and soft-tissue disruption.

Several techniques exist, including (but not limited to) distal clavicle resection, coracoacromical ligament transfer, AC or CC ligament repair, and CC ligament or dynamic muscle transfers. We prefer an anatomic coracoclavicular reconstruction (ACCR), which reconstructs the conoid and trapezoid ligaments separately using auto- or allograft through clavicular bone tunnels[3] (Figures 47-1 to 47-4). We do not resect the distal clavicle as part of this reconstruction because we believe the congruous bony surfaces impart stability to the reduced AC joint.

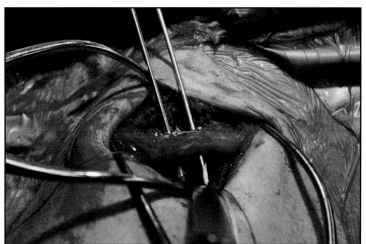

Figure 47-2. We prepare the clavicle by placing a guide pin 45 mm medial to the distal end of the clavicle and as posterior as possible, taking into consideration the space needed to not "blow out" the posterior cortical rim during reaming. This is where the reconstructed conoid ligament will be. We use a 6-mm cannulated reamer under power to create the tunnel. If there is a question of what size reamer to use, start with the smallest reamer necessary and ream in increasing increments as the clavicle tolerateses. We then disconnect the power driver and pull the reamer out manually to ensure that the tunnel is a perfect circle and not widened by uneven reaming. We repeat the same procedure for the trapezoid ligament, which is a more anterior structure than the conoid. We center this tunnel on the superior clavicle, approximately 15 mm lateral from the previous tunnel.

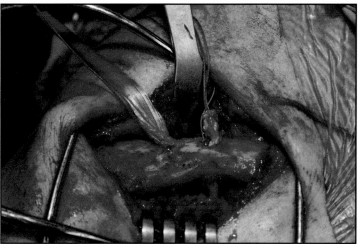

Figure 47-3. We position the graft so that the tail representing the conoid ligament is left 2 cm proud from the superior margin of the clavicle, whereas the long tail of the graft exits the trapezoid tunnel and will later be used to augment the AC joint repair if indicated.

Return to work or sport is determined with consideration of several factors. If a patient is treated nonoperatively, he may return to work or sport as symptoms allow. Patients treated with distal clavicle resection may begin range of motion (ROM) activities 1 to 2 days postoperatively. Strengthening starts at 4 to 6 weeks, with heavy lifting around 3 months. If a patient undergoes an ACCR, the he or she may begin supervised ROM in the supine position 7 to 10 days postoperatively. We will immobilize the patient in an abduction brace for 6 weeks to protect the healing graft. We allow active and active-assisted ROM from 6 to 12 weeks, and strengthening begins after 12 weeks. Patients may return to contact athletics or heavy labor at 6 months.

Figure 47-4. Next, we fold the short limb of the graft exiting the medial tunnel laterally and sew it to the base of the graft exiting the trapezoid tunnel in series. We then use the long limb exiting the lateral (trapezoid) tunnel laterally and loop it on top of the AC joint to augment the AC joint capsular repair. (Reprinted with permission from Arthrex, Inc, Naples, FL.)

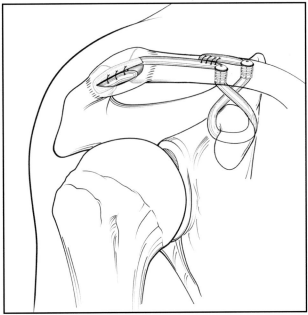

References

1. Phillips A, Smart C, Groom A. Acromioclavicular dislocation. *Clin Orthop Relat Res.* 1998;353:10-17.
2. Mazzocca AD, Arciero RA, Bicos J. Evaluation and treatment of acromioclavicular joint injuries. *Am J Sports Med.* 2007;35:316-329.
3. Mazzocca AD, Conway JE, Johnson S, Rios CG, Dumonski ML, Santangelo SA, Arciero RA. The anatomic coracoclavicular ligament reconstruction. *Oper Tech Sports Med.* 2004;12:56-61.

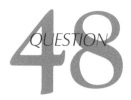

A WEIGHTLIFTER HAS OSTEOLYSIS OF THE DISTAL CLAVICLE ON A ZANCA VIEW RADIOGRAPH. THE PAIN HAS LIMITED THE ABILITY TO WORKOUT AND LIFT WEIGHTS. HOW DO YOU WORK-UP AND MANAGE A PATIENT WITH ACROMIOCLAVICULAR JOINT ARTHROSIS?

Justin W. Chandler, MD
Alex Creighton, MD

When we see a weightlifter with shoulder pain, we always have a clinical suspicion for osteolysis of the distal clavicle. Atraumatic osteolysis in weightlifting is felt to be due to cumulative subchondral stress fractures with a subsequent hypervascular response.[1] Osteolysis of the distal clavicle affects up to 28% of competitive weightlifters.[2] The diagnosis is suggested by history of repetitive use, most often in weightlifters, and physical examination with localized pain to palpation over the acromioclavicular (AC) joint, reproduction of symptoms at the AC joint with the cross-body adduction stress test, and internal rotation behind the back.

Radiographs of the shoulder, including a Zanca view of the AC joint, should be performed. The Zanca view is a 10-degree cephalic tilt anteroposterior (AP) of the AC joint with reduced penetration. This will allow you to see the osseous changes in the distal clavicle without overpentration and "burning out" the image at the distal clavicle. Otherwise, you may not see the characteristic radiologic findings of osteopenia,

Figure 48-1. Arthroscopic view from lateral portal of standard indirect approach.

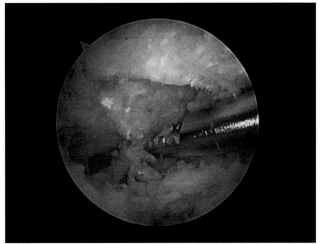

subchondral lysis and subchondral cysts[3] in the distal clavicle. We do not routinely use bone scans for this diagnosis, but technetium bone scans will demonstrate increased uptake at the distal clavicle. The differential diagnosis of AC joint pain includes other conditions associated with osteolysis, including hyperparathyroidism, rheumatoid arthritis, scleroderma, infection, and neoplasm.[1]

Treatment usually begins with conservative measures such as activity modification, nonsteroidal anti-inflammatory medicines, and intra-articular corticosteroid injections. Direct injections into the AC joint with a corticosteroid and lidocaine may be a useful diagnostic tool and may also provide some relief.

We find that a corticosteroid injection can decrease pain temporarily and may allow symptomatic relief. However, many times we find they do not provide long-term relief. This is due to the continued activity of the weightlifter. In the population of weightlifters behavior modification is often not an accepted treatment option.[2]

Surgical treatment consists of resection of the distal clavicle and was initially described as an open procedure in 1941.[4] This procedure has been shown to be a reliable treatment for painful AC joint pathology refractory to nonoperative treatment.[5] More recently, arthroscopic distal clavicle resection has been advocated, offering the advantages of decreased morbidity, fewer postoperative restrictions on motion, earlier return to normal activity, and improved cosmesis.[6] The arthroscopic approach may also protect the important superior capsule of the AC joint.

Two methods of arthroscopic distal clavicle resection have been described: a direct superior approach and an indirect subacromial approach. The indirect approach utilizes standard posterior, anterior, and lateral subacromial portals (Figure 48-1). The lateral portal is initially used to assess the depth of the distal clavicle resection; a burr is used through the anterior portal (directly in line with the acromioclavicular joint) to resect the distal clavicle, with the arthroscope in the lateral portal.[4]

In osteolysis of the distal clavicle, we prefer the direct superior approach. The direct superior approach utilizes 2 portals—the posterosuperior portal 1 cm posterior to the AC joint and the anterosuperior portal 1 cm anterior to the AC joint. A resection of approximately 8 to 10 mm is performed through anterior and posterior portals, alternating arthroscope and burr positions (Figure 48-2).

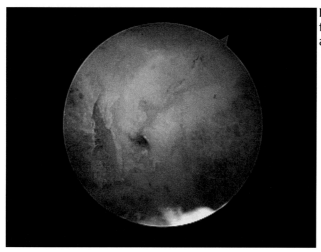

Figure 48-2. Arthroscopic view from anterior portal utilizing direct approach.

In a recent randomized prospective study, Charron and colleagues[7] compared the direct and indirect approaches for distal clavicle resection in athletes. Both groups demonstrated significant improvement in clinical outcome scores at a minimum 2-year follow-up. However, the direct approach group had significantly higher scores in the American Shoulder and Elbow Surgeons (ASES) and Athletic Shoulder Scoring System scores at week 2 ($P < 0.001$), week 6 ($P < 0.001$), and final follow-up ($P < 0.001$). The direct group also demonstrated significantly faster return to sports at mean of 21 days, compared to mean of 42 days in the indirect group ($P < 0.001$).

Auge and Fischer[1] used the direct arthroscopic approach in 10 consecutive weightlifters with atraumatic osteolysis of the distal clavicle. Average time to return to weightlifting was 3.2 days and the athletes were back to their preoperative weight-training program at a mean 9.1 days. All athletes remained asymptomatic through an average follow-up of 18.7 months.

Zawadsky and colleagues[5] studied long-term results of the direct arthroscopic approach in 41 shoulders with average follow-up of 6.2 years. They had 93% good or excellent results with no significant compromise in function and either slight or no postoperative pain. The 3 patients who failed the arthroscopic procedure had sustained direct trauma to the AC joint in either a fall or motor vehicle collision.

Atraumatic osteolysis of the distal clavicle is an uncommon cause of shoulder pain, but in the subpopulation of competitive weightlifters and arm-lifting athletes, it is quite prevalent. It can cause significant pain and limit the athlete's performance. Nonoperative treatment options may be successful if the athlete is willing to modify his activity level, but arthroscopic distal clavicle resection provides a reliable method of treatment with early return to activity, minimal morbidity, and excellent cosmesis.

References

1. Auge WK 2nd, Fischer RA. Arthroscopic distal clavicle resection for isolated atraumatic osteolysis in weight lifters. *Am J Sports Med.* 1998;26:189-192.
2. Scavenius M, Iversen BF. Nontraumatic clavicular osteolysis in weight lifters. *Am J Sports Med.* 1992;20:463-467.

3. Beals RK, Sauser DD. Nontraumatic disorders of the clavicle. *J Am Acad Orthop Surg.* 2006;14:205-214.
4. Mumford EB. Acromioclavicular dislocation: a new operative treatment. *J Bone Joint Surg Am.* 1941;23:79-801.
5. Zawadsky M, Marra G, Wiater JM, Levine WN, Pollock RG, Flatow EL, Bigliani LU. Osteolysis of the distal clavicle: long-term results of arthroscopic resection. *Arthroscopy.* 2000;16:600-605.
6. Gartsman GM. Arthroscopic resection of the acromioclavicular joint. *Am J Sports Med.* 1993;21:71-77.
7. Charron KM, Schepsis AA, Voloshin I. Arthroscopic distal clavicle resection in athletes: a prospective comparison of the direct and indirect approach. *Am J Sports Med.* 2007;35:53-58.

SECTION X

STIFFNESS QUESTION

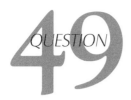

WHAT ARE THE INDICATIONS FOR MANIPULATION UNDER ANESTHESIA VERSUS ARTHROSCOPIC RELEASE IN A PATIENT WITH STIFFNESS AFTER ROTATOR CUFF REPAIR? AND WHEN DO YOU CONSIDER OPERATIVE INTERVENTION IN A PATIENT WITH IDIOPATHIC ADHESIVE CAPSULITIS?

Michael Freehill, MD

The patient with a stiff shoulder following a rotator cuff repair, particularly one done arthroscopically, has become more challenging recently. There seems to be a wave of enthusiasm for a decelerated physical therapy program to allow for potential greater healing of the rotator cuff repair performed arthroscopically. A recent study indicated that patients who actually had greater earlier stiffness had a higher rate of intact rotator cuff repairs than those who were nonstiff following arthroscopic repair.[1] Decelerated rehabilitation programs can lead to the potential of early stiffness following arthroscopic repair. In a study of complications after arthroscopic repair, stiffness was the most common complication recognized, but was noted to respond to conservative management in the majority of cases.[2]

The duration of conservative care is quite variable depending on whether the cause of adhesive capsulitis (stiffness) is a primary or idiopathic etiology, or a secondary cause such as post-traumatic injury or operative intervention. Griggs and colleagues[3] indicated significant improvements at the mid term (6 to 12 weeks) of conservative treatment with 90% satisfaction at final follow up (12 to 41 months). There were however, appreciable motion and functional deficits when compared to the unaffected shoulder.

This is one potential reason why there is such confusion on how to truly treat the frozen shoulder. In general, if physical therapy has failed to yield functional outcome in which the patient has restoration of function of the shoulder with 80 to 90% of the contralateral unaffected shoulder within 6 to 12 months, operative intervention should be strongly considered. This is particularly the case in patients who have a secondary cause such as a rotator cuff repair. Furthermore, if the patient is truly dissatisfied with the progress of physical therapy within the first 3 to 6 months of care and has basically plateaued in his functional improvement, the decision to perform operative intervention may be hastened.

After operative intervention has been determined as the course of treatment, the next decision becomes whether or not to perform a manipulation under anesthesia or an arthroscopic release. In the case of a patient who presents with stiffness following an arthroscopic rotator cuff repair, it is this author's opinion that manipulation under anesthesia should not be performed under any circumstances. Any surgeon who has put an arthroscope in the patient's shoulder after a forceful manipulation knows that there is significant soft-tissue damage, as evidence by the hemarthrosis that is usually encountered. In addition, there is a risk for potential damage to the rotator cuff, particularly one that has been recently repaired. I recommend an elective arthroscopic capsular release focusing on the areas identified during the examination under anesthesia that require specific attention. The glenohumeral capsule, the rotator interval, and the subacromial space can all be involved in the pathologic process after rotator cuff repairs.

If the patient has significant restrictions in external rotation, then the coracohumeral ligament and rotator interval will need to be addressed. When forward elevation and abduction is also limited, then attention needs to be turned to the anterior/anteroinferior capsule and axillary recess region. A significant posterior capsule contracture may be required circumferential release will be required in this case to include the posterior capsule. This author tends to avoid the area from 5 to 7 o'clock in the axillary recess when performing a capsular release. Typically, following a near circumferential arthroscopic release, with the exception of this region, a very gentle manipulation in abduction can be performed to achieve the remaining motion to allow for full restoration of range of motion (ROM). An electrocautery probe or radiofrequency probe can be utilized to perform the arthroscopic release if the surgeon is comfortable with this instrumentation. Soft-tissue biters can also be used to perform the release, but typically takes a greater time period.

The debridement of any scar tissue or synovitis should be performed concurrently with the arthroscopic release. In patients who have had a previous rotator cuff repair, a strong consideration for an extra-articular release in the subacromial and subdeltoid space should be taken into consideration. Diagnostic arthroscopy and bursectomy with release of any subacromial and subdeltoid adhesions can be performed relatively easily via arthroscopic technique.

The treatment of a patient who has idiopathic adhesive capsulitis tends to be conservative compared to secondary adhesive capsulitis. Recent studies have demonstrated that approximately 90% of the time patients with idiopathic adhesive capsulitis, including those who are diabetic, will achieve near full functional recovery within 12 months of the onset of nonoperative management.[4] My treatment algorithm typically includes a fluoroscopically guided glenohumeral corticosteroid injection in addition to a home exercise program focusing on active and active assisted ROM. A stretching program emphasizing elevation, external rotation (ER), and internal rotation (IR) is instituted. If they fail to achieve a functional ROM within 12 months, have plateau in their functional recovery for a minimum of 3 months, or they have moved beyond the painful phase of adhesive capsulitis, then I consider operative intervention.

Overall, the decision to treat a frozen shoulder conservatively or operatively depends on numerous factors. Comorbid conditions such as diabetes or cardiovascular disease and the patient's smoking status should be taken into consideration. This author tends to treat secondary causes such as postoperative stiffness more aggressively than an idiopathic etiology. In general, if the patient fails to achieve functional improvements over a course of 3 to 4 months of conservative management, consideration for operative intervention should be taken into account. This author is not a fan of manipulation under anesthesia or any other fancier techniques such as hydroplasty. A careful examination under anesthesia and any selective controlled arthroscopic capsular release, I believe, brings the best potential outcome from a functional standpoint. An arthroscopic approach also affords the surgeon a chance to address any concomitant pathologies that may be causing symptoms in a patient, such as acromioclavicular (AC) joint arthrosis, subacromial impingement, and biceps and/or rotator cuff pathology. An arthroscopic capsular release also avoids potential complications such as extensive soft-tissue damage or in the case of elderly patients, possible fracture that can occur during the manipulation.

References

1. Occousti KG, Parson B, Gladstone JN, et al. Does slower rehabilitation after arthroscopic rotator cuff repair lead to stiffness? SS-22. Presented at Arthroscopy Association for North America 26th Annual Meeting, April 26-29, 2007, San Francisco, CA.
2. Brislin KJ, Field LD, Savoie FH. Complications after arthroscopic rotator cuff repair. *Arthroscopy*. 2007; 23:124-128.
3. Griggs S. Idiopathic adhesive capsulitis: a prospective functional outcome study of nonoperative treatment. *J Bone Joint Surg*. 2000; 82:1398.
4. Levine WN, Kashyap CP, Bak SF, Ahmad CS, Blaine TA, Bigliani LU. Nonoperative management of idiopathic adhesive capsulitis. *J Shoulder Elbow Surg*. 2007;16(5):569-573.

INDEX

Printed in the United States
by Baker & Taylor Publisher Services